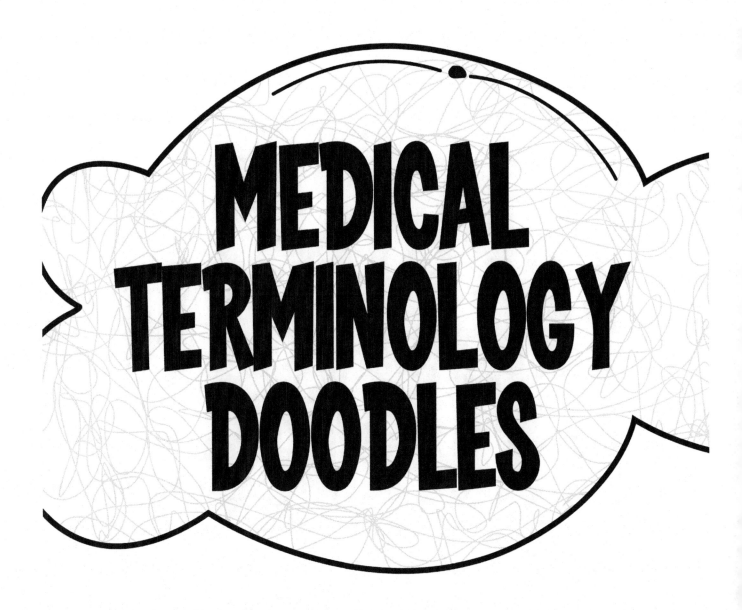

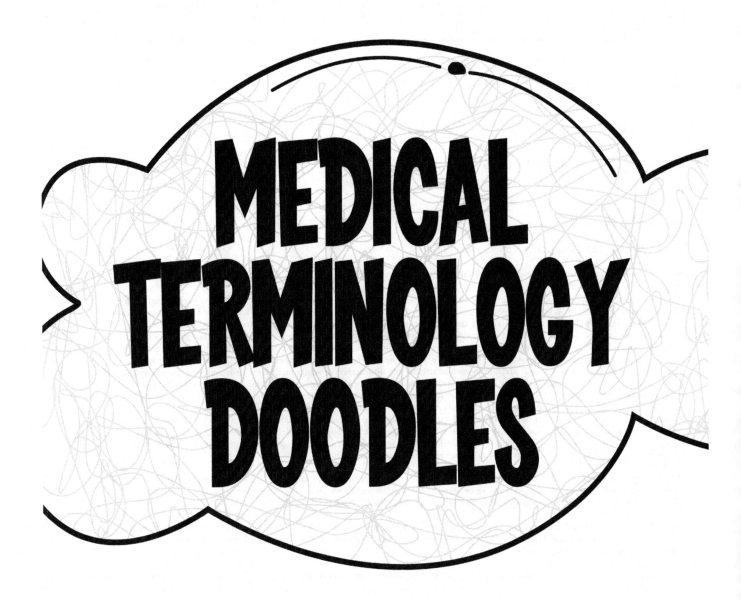

MEDICAL TERMINOLOGY DOODLES

Karen Sladyk, PhD, OTR, FAOTA
Westfield State University
Westfield, Massachusetts

Illustrator
Giancarlo Romeo

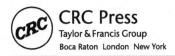

CRC Press
Taylor & Francis Group
Boca Raton London New York

CRC Press is an imprint of the
Taylor & Francis Group, an **informa** business

Medical Terminology Doodles includes ancillary materials specifically available for faculty use. Included are medical terminology tests. Please visit http://www.routledge.com/9781630914806 to obtain access.

Cover Artist: Lori Shields

First published 2020 by SLACK Incorporated

Published 2024 by CRC Press
2385 NW Executive Center Drive, Suite 320, Boca Raton FL 33431

and by CRC Press
4 Park Square, Milton Park, Abingdon, Oxon, OX14 4RN

CRC Press is an imprint of Taylor & Francis Group, LLC

© 2020 Taylor & Francis Group, LLC

Dr. Karen Sladyk has no financial or proprietary interest in the materials presented herein.

Library of Congress Cataloging-in-Publication Data

Names: Sladyk, Karen, 1958- author. | Romeo, Giancarlo, illustrator.

Title: Medical terminology doodles / Karen Sladyk ; illustrator, Giancarlo
  Romeo.

Description: Thorofare, NJ : SLACK Incorporated, [2020]

Identifiers: LCCN 2019041521 | ISBN 9781630914806 (paperback)

Subjects: MESH: Terminology as Topic | Medicine | Terminology | Examination
  Question

Classification: LCC R123 | NLM W 15 | DDC 610.1/4--dc23

LC record available at https://lccn.loc.gov/2019041521

ISBN:9781630914806(pbk)
ISBN:9781003525059(ebk)

DOI: 10.1201/9781003525059

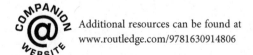

Additional resources can be found at
www.routledge.com/9781630914806

Contents

Acknowledgments . . . . *vii*

About the Author. . . . . *ix*

Introduction. . . . . *xi*

MEDICAL TERMINOLOGY DOODLES

A. 1		M 140
B. 38		N. 156
C. 48		O. 164
D. 74		P. 175
E. 86		Q. 213
F. 100		R. 214
G. 106		S. 225
H. 115		T. 244
I. 123		U. 255
J. 129		V. 259
K. 130		X. 264
L. 131		Z. 266

Exercises. 267

Answer Key 273

Medical Terminology Lists 279

Medical Terminology Doodles includes ancillary materials specifically available for faculty use. Included are medical terminology tests. Please visit http://www.routledge.com/9781630914806 to obtain access.

Acknowledgments

I am forever thankful to the people of SLACK Incorporated for their support, attention to detail, and passion. As I believe gratitude is essential for creativity to grow, I am especially thankful for their warm friendship. In particular, thank you to Stephanie Arasim Portnoy, Jennifer Kilpatrick, Mary Sasso, Brien Cummings, Allegra Tiver, Thomas Cavallaro, Lori Shields, and Emily Densten.

About the Author

Karen Sladyk, PhD, OTR, FAOTA teaches health sciences at Westfield State University in Westfield, Massachusetts. She is a graduate of the occupational therapy program at Eastern Michigan University. Karen holds a masters in community health education from Southern Connecticut State University and PhD in adult and vocational education from the University of Connecticut. When not in the classroom, she enjoys travel and crafting, both of which provide her with gratitude for living a life of meaning.

Introduction

Welcome to a different way to learn medical terminology, with movement! Flashcards are nice, and practice lists are good, but **moving** is better. This book suggests that a multi-sensory approach to learning words is better than traditional methods.

THE POWER OF A DOODLE

Doodling your vocabulary terms helps you better picture the meaning of the word. Drawing the vocabulary word helps form a permanent link in your mind by connecting several sections of your brain with the associated term. Drawing doodles reminds you of the meaning of the word root and helps you learn the word root kinesthetically. After all, we do not take tests with flashcards, we write the answer. It makes sense to learn material in the way we have to use it. Flashcards often fail students because they can "see" the word on the card but cannot remember to "see" the answer. This book covers the 266 most popular medical terms that will get you started in your health care occupation.

Doodle suggestions are made for each term in this book, but you can personalize your learning by assigning meaning to the term yourself. The word root will have a "consider this ..." suggestion; however, you should do a doodle that has meaning to you. Sometimes it is impossible to draw a concept everyone can understand, so the suggestions are just that, suggestions. The doodler must make meaning of the word root. You may want to consider rewriting the word root in a style that suggests the meaning, such as large squiggly lines for large intestines. Consider doodling the "you may already know" term as another way to reinforce the word root. These terms are related to the word root on each page. Also, reinforce your doodle by saying the root and meaning while you doodle.

MEDICAL TERMINOLOGY FOUNDATIONS

Before you can begin to understand complicated medical words, it is useful to understand how the words are put together. Medical terminology generally follows some basic rules. Once you master these rules, breaking down very long words, such as electroencephalogram (record of the electrical activity of the brain), becomes easy. Most medical words are made up of **word parts**. These include:

- Word roots
- Prefixes (before the word root)
- Suffixes (after the word root)
- Connecting vowel (between two word roots)

An example of how this works in real life includes the words **play**, **player**, and **replay**. **Play** is the word root, the foundation to the word. The suffix -**er** is added to mean the person at play. In replay, **re**- is the prefix meaning to repeat the play again. Now, let's examine some basic medical words. **Arthritis** and **hepatitis** are two medical terms familiar to most people. **Arthr** means joint and **hepat** means liver. The suffix -**itis** means inflammation. So, arthritis is inflammation of the joints and hepatitis is inflammation of the liver. Generally speaking, the way to assign meaning to the word is to start with the suffix first. Arthritis becomes inflammation of the joints instead of joint inflammation.

Some of the most commonly used medical terminology suffixes include:

- -logy (study of)
- -logist (one who studies)

Medical terminology breaks down to the study of terms, and you are a medical terminologist. Knowing these two suffixes alone will aid you in understanding almost every medical specialty.

Connecting vowels are sometimes called **combining vowels**. More often than not, the connecting vowel is the letter o. **Arthropathy** is an example of the connecting vowel between the word roots **arthr** (joints) and **pathy** (disease). Arthropathy means disease of the joints.

There are two medical terminology meanings that have multiple suffixes. These can be initially confusing, but after you have seen words that use "pertaining to" and "condition of," it will make better sense than the list here. It is handy if you know about the existence of these suffixes before you start to study medical terminology. These are listed here:

- **Pertaining to**: -ac, -al, -an, -ar, -eal, -ic, -ive, -ous
- **Condition of**: -ia, -ism, -osis

SPELLING HINTS

- Medical words do not always have a prefix, but typically have a suffix.
- Do not use a connecting vowel if the suffix begins with a vowel.
- Do not use a connecting vowel between a prefix and a word root.
- When unsure of which connecting vowel to use, use the letter o, as it is the most common.

MEMORIZING HINTS

In your chosen medical career, you will often hear about evidence-based practice. Evidence-based practice means using the most current research to guide your treatment decisions (Brahler & Walker, 2008). As a health care provider, this means your learning never ends and you are expected to be able to read current research on assessment and treatment news. You already know that you need to understand medical terminology to read medical journals and research papers, but what does the research say about learning medical terminology? The following hints are based on the research in memorizing things like medical terminology.

A few word roots at a time over a long time is better than an all-night cram session. Every student knows a little content over time is better than trying to stuff 250 word roots in your head over night, yet time management often appears to interfere with this approach. The real issue may not be time management but rather breaking ineffective, but well-ingrained, preferred studying techniques (Glenn, 2009).

An organized learning area will help you stay focused, but do not let the organizing take more time than the studying. Jungert and Rosander (2009) found the learning environment was by far the most common strategy used by graduate students when sitting down to study content material. The learning area was influenced by the learners' approach to studying and may or may not have included group-peer studying, but an organized learning area can only facilitate the preferred study methods.

Colored pencils vs. lead pencils? Polychrome (colored pencils) vs. monochrome (lead pencil) is up to you. You can always add colored pencils over your lead pencil doodles. Pencils will not leak through to the next page like some markers will. You may not have used crayons in a long time, but they offer a million color choices, are inexpensive, and also do not leak through to the next page. But the bottom line is, simply by reading this paragraph, you likely learned that the word root chrome means color.

Practice medical terminology in different environments so the retrieval of the information is not dependent on the place you learned. McDaniel, Howard, and Einstein (2009) and McDaniel, Wildman, and Anderson (2012) stated that students needed to close the book and actively try to recall as much as possible either in written or spoken word. Rereading note cards defeats the true learning of the text and leads to a false confidence. Karpicke and Roediger (2010) found rereading information leads to a sense of familiarity and confidence, but when in a testing situation, the learner was unable to reconstruct the knowledge. Also, start integrating the terms into your everyday conversations.

Besides the kinesthetic learning of doodling, use auditory and visual techniques you like. Karpicke and Roediger (2010) showed learners who read passages from a book out loud did far better in recall than those who read the passages silently. Beaton et al. (2005) suggested linking the word root to another word that either sounds similar or for which an image can be visualized. Doodling helps form that image. Although there are suggested doodles on each page, there is intentionally large blank areas for the learner to doodle their own interpretation of the word root.

Make practice exams to take and share with friends so you can take different styles of tests (McDaniel et al., 2012). Every person writes tests in different styles, which test not only content, but problem solving as well. Each test maker organizes information differently than another, so each test will have different selection of content and will help the learner make new associations, thereby diversifying the content (Jairam & Kiewra, 2009).

Find comfort in knowing millions of health care students have mastered medical terminology before you and many will follow you as well.

STUDY HINTS

- Buy a medical terminology dictionary.
- Make a study peer group to share ideas and techniques.
- Make your own flashcards and quiz yourself.
- Wall posters made out of freezer paper or newsprint allow you to think and draw **big**. Freezer paper is particularly useful because the plastic coating on the back of the paper prevents permanent marker from leaking through to the wall but lets you write in bright colors. The front of freezer paper is bright white and porous to markers. You will find freezer paper in your local grocery store, typically on the shelf near the tin foil and plastic wrap.
- Apps, such as Quizlet, and audio recordings made using note taking or recording apps on your phone can be used in your study group.
- Develop your own worksheets that combine word roots, prefixes, and suffixes. Share with friends in your study group. Use the word root in a sentence that has meaning to you. At the end of this book, you will find a condensed listing of the word roots covered in this text. Use this list to quiz yourself, make your own tests, or write sentences practicing the meaning of each word root.
- Make a game night by using a commercially available game board and substituting your own cards. All studying goes better with a game, snacks, and prizes.
- Remember, the most important part is to doodle what is important to you, not necessarily what we suggest.
- You have to learn medical terminology if you want to become an expert health care provider, so you might as well have fun doing it. Enjoy!

REFERENCES

Beaton, A., Gruneberg, M., Hyde, C., Shufflebottom, A., & Sykes, R. (2005). Facilitation of receptive and productive foreign vocabulary learning using keyword method: The role of image quality. *Memory, 13*(5), 458-471. doi: 10.1080/09658210444000395

Brahler, C. J., & Walker, D. (2008). Learning scientific and medical terminology with a mnemonic strategy using an illogical association technique. *Advances in Physiology Education, 32*, 219-224. doi: 10.1152/advance.00083.2007

Glenn, D. (2009). Close the book. Recall. Write it down. *Chronicle of Higher Education, 55*(34), A1.

Jairam, D., & Kiewra, K. A. (2009). An investigation of the SOAR study method. *Journal of Advanced Academics, 20*(4), 602-629.

Jungert, T., & Rosander, M. (2009). Relationships between students' strategies for influencing their study environment and their strategic approach to studying. *Studies in Higher Education, 34*(2), 139-152. doi: 10.1080/03075070802596970

Karpicke, J. D., & Roediger, H. L. (2010). Is expanding retrieval a superior method for learning text materials? *Memory & Cognition, 38*, 116-124. doi: 10.3758/MC.38.1.116

McDaniel, M. A., Howard, D. C., & Einstein, G. O. (2009). The read-recite-review study strategy: Effective and portable. *Psychological Science, 20*(4), 516-522. doi: 10.111/j.1467-9280.2009.02325.x

McDaniel, M. A., Wildman, K. M., & Anderson, J. L. (2012). Using quizzes to enhance summative-assessment performance in a web-based class: An experimental study. *Journal of Applied Research in Memory and Cognition, 1*, 18-26. doi: 10.1016/j.jarma.2011.10.001

Consider a doodle of
a rocket ship without oxygen

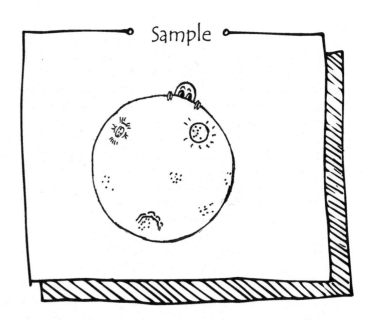

Sample

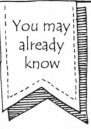

Anemia below normal red blood cells, **Anarchy** without government or law,
Anoxia no oxygen, **Anesthesia** loss of feeling or sensation, **Alogia** inability to
speak due to mental deficiency

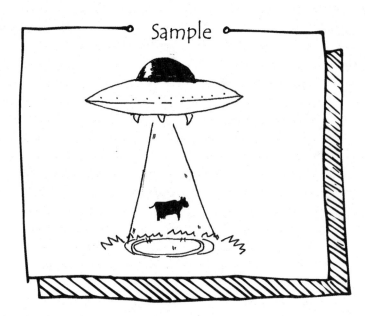

Sample

Consider a doodle of
an alien being abducted

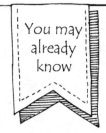
Abnormal different from what is considered normal, **Abatement** stopping
something from happening, **Abrasion** rubbing away, **Abduction** taken away

Consider a doodle of
an abnormal abdomen

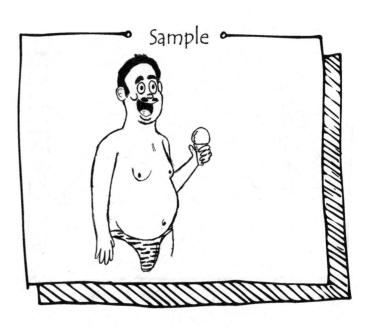

Sample

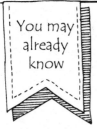

You may
already
know

Abdominal pertaining to the abdomen, **Abdominohysterectomy** hysterectomy
through an abdominal incision, **Celiotomy** surgical incision into the abdomen

Consider a doodle of
a bottle of acid

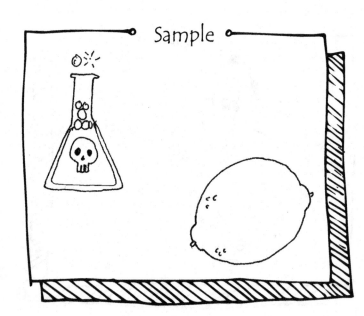

Sample

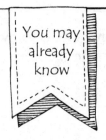

You may
already
know

Acidity how sour something is, **Acidosis** condition of acidic kidneys or lungs

Consider a doodle of
an acoustic guitar

Sample

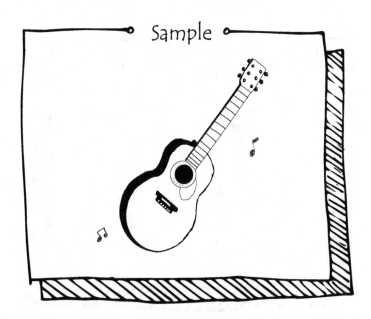

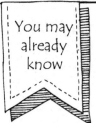

You may
already
know

Acoustic guitar an instrument, **Acousmatamnesia** failure to recall sounds

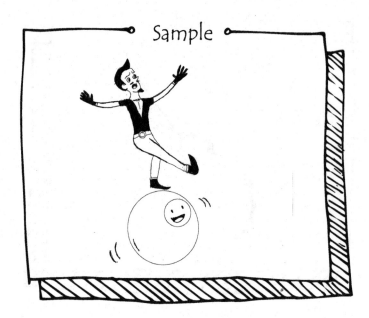

Sample

Consider a doodle of
an acrobat on top of a ball

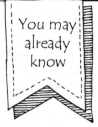

You may
already
know

Acrobat performs high in the air, **Acrophobia** fear of heights, **Acroagnosis** lack
of sensory recognition of an extremity, **Acromegaly** enlarged nose, fingers,
or toes

Consider a doodle of
needles in letters: A, C, U

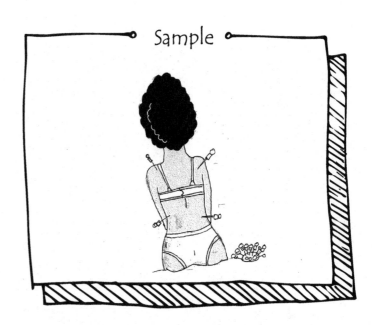

Sample

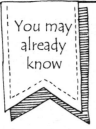

You may
already
know

Acute sharp symptoms, **Acupuncture** alternative treatment involving needles,
Aculalia severe nonsense speech, **Acus** needle-like process,
Acuminate sharp point

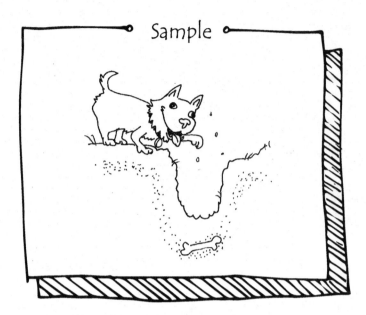

Sample

Consider a doodle of
a dog nearly reaching
a bone

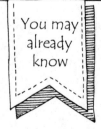

You may
already
know

Ad hoc committee formed in addition to normal committees for a specific
purpose, **Adduction** toward the median plane

Consider a doodle of
letters made of fat:
A, D, I, P

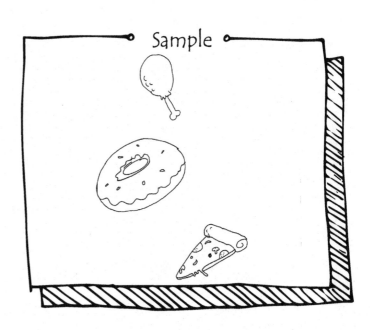

Sample

Adipose fat animal, **Adiposis** obesity, **Adipocele** hernia containing fat

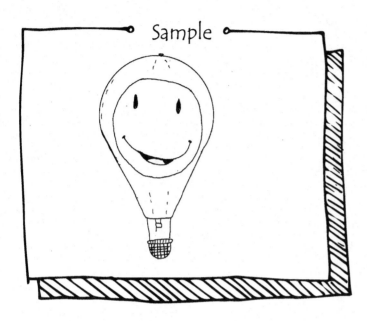

Sample

Consider a doodle of
a hot air balloon

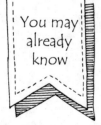

You may
already
know

Aerosol particles suspended in air, **Aeronaut** one who operates an airship or
balloon, **Aerophagia** habitual swallowing of air

Consider a doodle of
a boy waking a bear

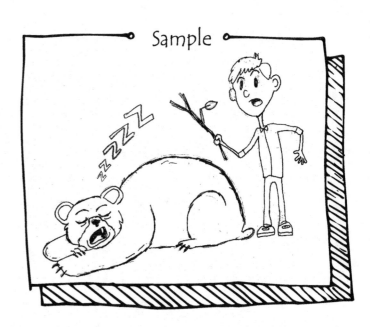

Sample

You may
already
know

Agitate move back and forth rapidly, **Agitated** feeling restless

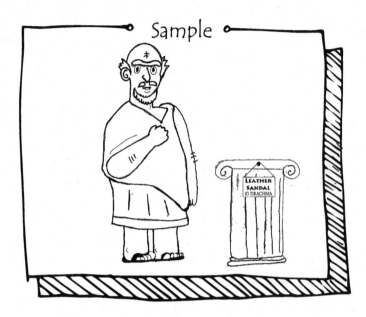

Sample

Consider a doodle of
Caesar in the marketplace

Consider a doodle of
a white lab rat

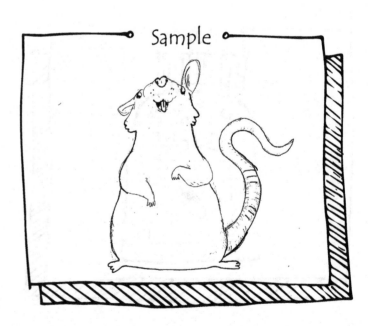

Sample

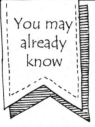

Albino animal any animal without pigmentation in the eyes, skin, or hair,
Albino skin type congenital absence of normal pigmentation

Consider a doodle of
a medicine bottle

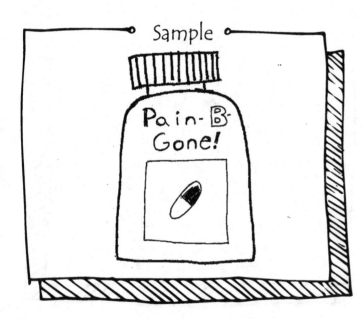

Sample

Pain-B-
Gone!

You may
already
know

Analgesic compound to relieve pain, such as aspirin, **Algesia** sensitive to pain,
Algesimetry measurement of pain sensitivity

Consider a doodle of
a person in pain

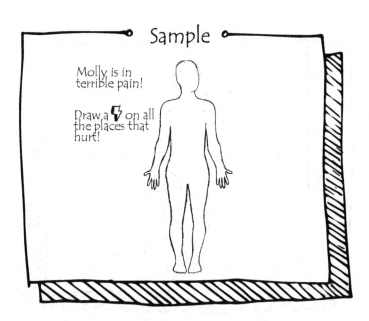

Sample

Molly is in
terrible pain!

Draw a ⚡ on all
the places that
hurt!

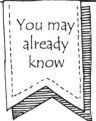

Fibromyalgia painful condition, **Cephalalgia** headache

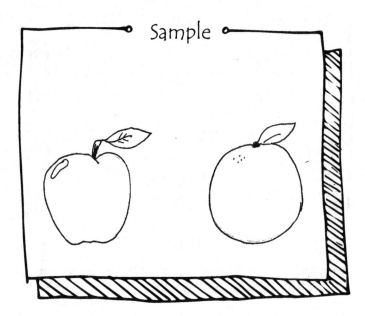

Sample

Consider a doodle
comparing apples
to oranges

Alloy different metals mixed together, **Alloplastic adaptation** ability to
manipulate the environment

Consider a doodle of
Ami swinging with
her parents

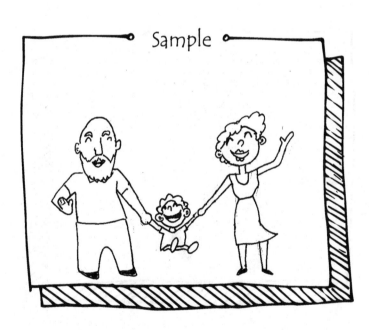

Sample

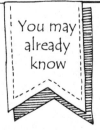

Ambidextrous using both hands, **Ambivalence** on both sides of like and dislike; conflicting emotional attitudes toward goals, **Ambisexual** characteristic of both genders, **Ambiopia** double vision

Consider a doodle of
a kid taking a walk

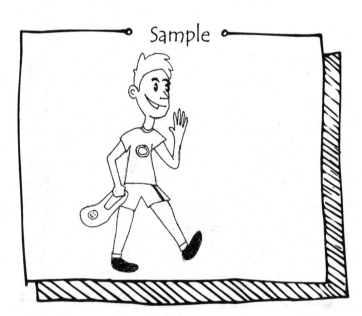

Sample

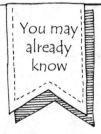

You may
already
know

Ambulance a vehicle used to deliver a medical patient, **Ambulate** to walk

Consider a doodle of
an analogy

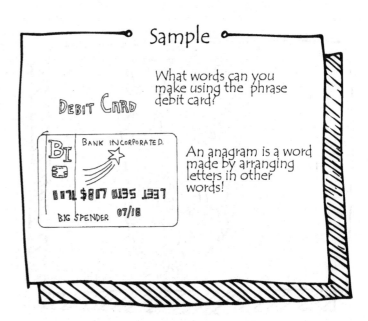

Sample

What words can you
make using the phrase
debit card?

DEBIT CARD

BANK INCORPORATED.
BI

007L $807 0135 1337

BIG SPENDER   07/18

An anagram is a word
made by arranging
letters in other
words!

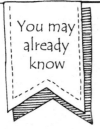

You may
already
know

Analysis exam by breaking into parts, **Analogue** of the same parts,
Analogy associate two like words, **Anasarca** massive edema,
Anaphylactic shock to have an excessive reaction to a substance,
Anaphia loss of touch

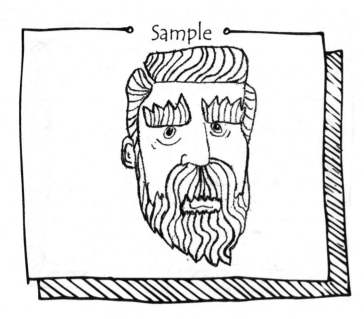

Sample

Consider a doodle of
letters in a man's beard:
A, N, D, R, O

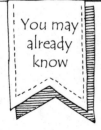

Android man-like machine, **Androgynous** having both male and female
characteristics

Consider a doodle of
a snake with a sac

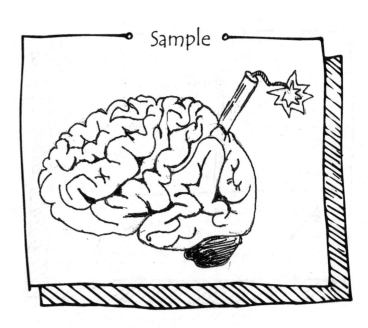

Sample

You may
already
know

Aneurysm sac breaking and bleeding, **Aneurysmoplasty** repair of an artery
affected by aneurysm

Consider a doodle of
a sea vessel named Angie

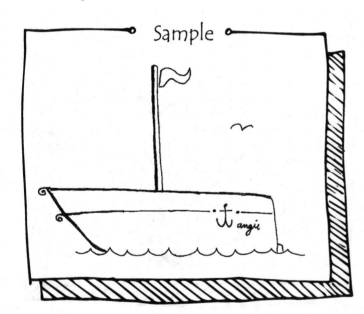

Sample

You may
already
know

Angiogram common measure of heart function, **Angioplasty** surgical opening
of heart arteries using a catheter with balloon or laser

ankyl/o   stiff, crooked, bent, looped around

Consider a doodle of
a dinosaur with big ankles

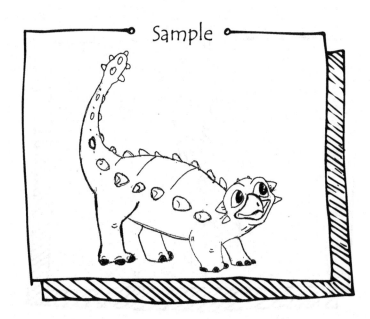
Sample

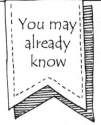**Anklet** jewelry on your ankle, **Ankylosis** fused or frozen joint

Sample

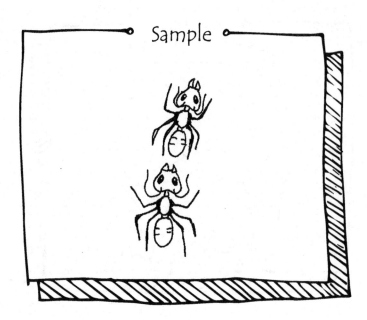

Consider a doodle of
ants marching in front of
each other

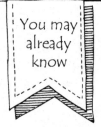

You may
already
know

Anterior toward the front, **Ancestors** family in history, **Anterolateral** in front or
to the side

Consider a doodle of
protesters

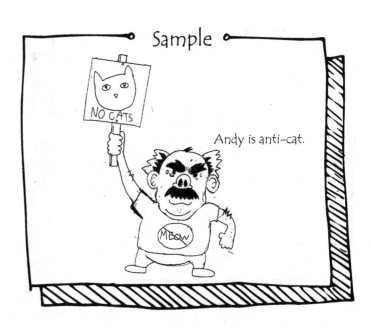

Sample

Andy is anti-cat.

Antibullying against intimidation, **Contraindicated** against advice,
Antidepressant preventing or relieving depression, **Antidiuretic** suppression
of urine

Consider a doodle of
an aquarium full of letters:
A, Q, U, E

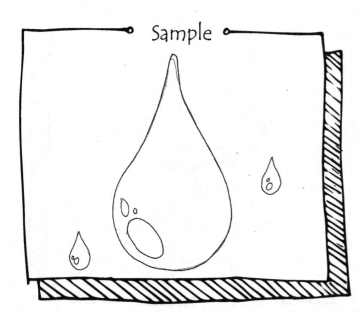

Sample

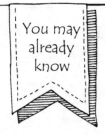

Aqueduct roadway of water, **Aquaphobia** fear of water, **Aqueous** watery

Consider a doodle of
a victory (first place) arch

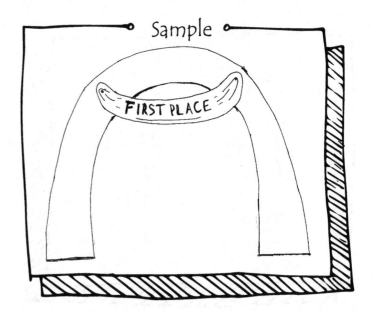

Sample

FIRST PLACE

You may
already
know

Archrival number one enemy, **Archetype** original idea,
Archencephalon primitive brain

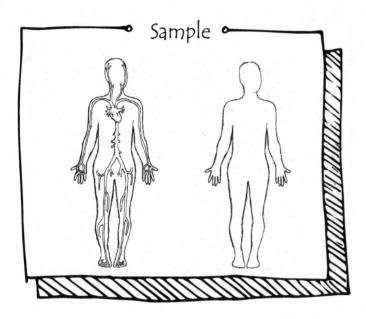

Sample

Consider a doodle of
an artery system

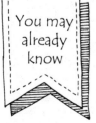

You may
already
know

Artery vessel that carries blood away from the heart, **Arteriospasm** spasm of
an artery

Consider a doodle of
crabs

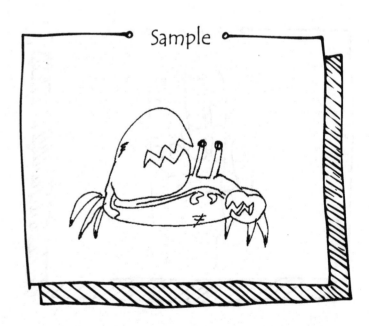

Sample

You may
already
know

Arthritis inflammation of the joints, **Arthropod** jointed animal, such as a crab,
Arthroscopy examining inside the joint with an instrument

Consider a doodle of
jointed puppets

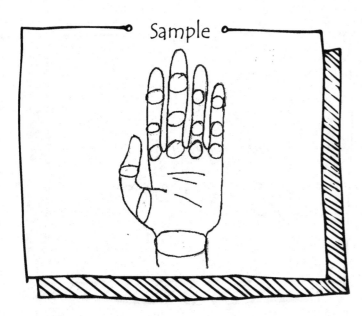

Sample

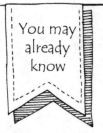

Articulate united by a joint, **Articulation** the place of union of a joint

Consider a doodle of
a vacuum that inhales

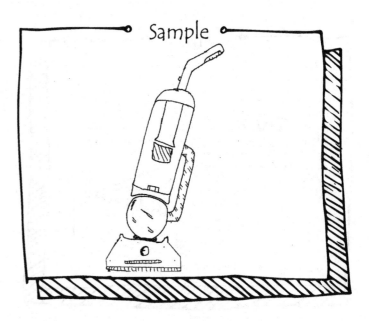

Sample

Aspirated breathing food particles into the airway, **Aspiration** inhaled substances, such as saliva, food, or other liquids or solids, into the lungs

Sample

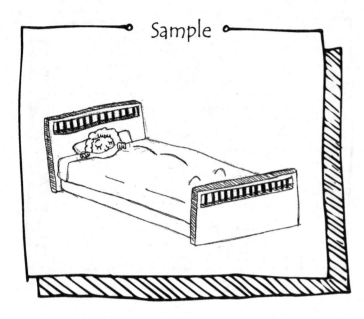

Consider a doodle of
Annie sleeping

You may
already
know

Anesthesia chemicals that put you to sleep for surgery, **Asthenopia** easy fatigue
of the eyes, **Asthenic** condition of weak strength

- -

Consider a doodle of
letters made of fat:
A, T, H, E, R

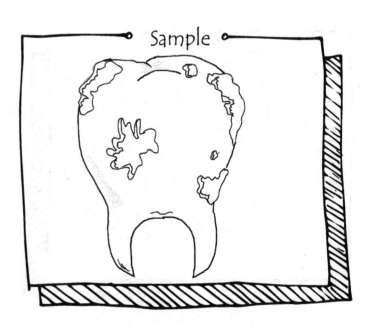

Sample

You may
already
know

Atheromatosis diffused arterial disease

Consider a doodle of
headphones

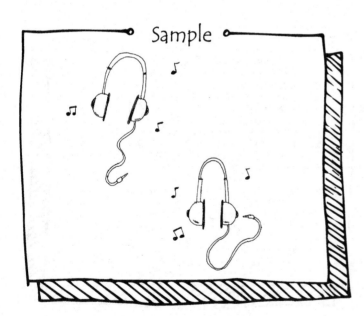

Sample

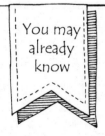

You may
already
know

Audio sound, **Audiovisual** made for both sight and hearing,
Audiometry measurement of hearing, **Dysaudia** impaired hearing

- -

Consider a doodle of
an ear

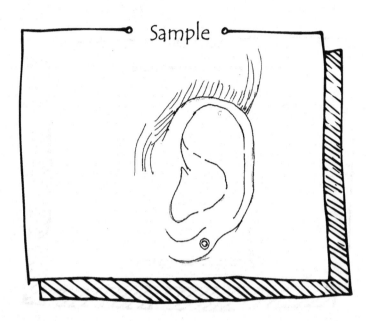

Sample

You may
already
know

Aural sense of hearing, **Auripuncture** surgical puncture of the tympanic
membrane, **Auriscope** an instrument used to examine the ear

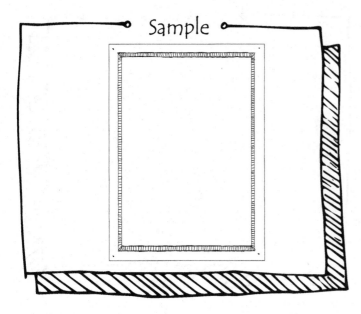
Sample

Consider a doodle of
a person looking at
him- or herself

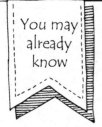
You may
already
know

Automobile car, **Autonomic** without voluntary control,
Autohemotherapy treatment using the patient's own blood, **Autoplasty** tissue
from one region to another, **Autotrophic** self-nourishing

Consider a doodle of
a cord spelling aux

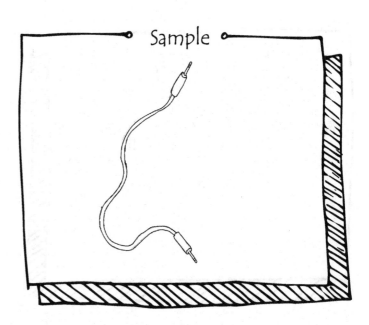

Sample

Auxin plant hormone that stimulates growth, **Auxodrome** a child's course of
growth chart, **Auxometry** measurement of the rate of growth

Consider a doodle of
germs

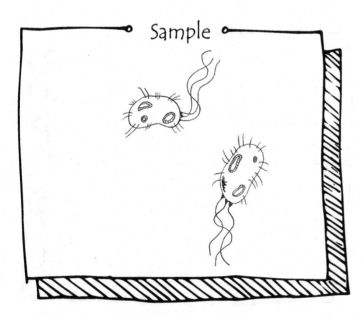

Sample

Bacteria germ causing disease, **Bacteriogenic** bacterial in origin, **Bacterid** skin
eruption from an infection elsewhere

Consider a doodle of
a walking sign

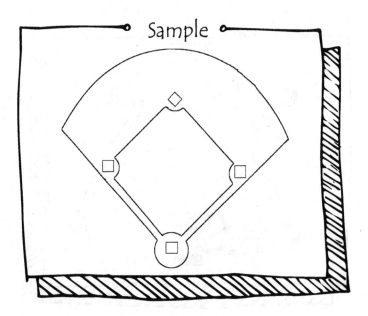

Sample

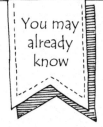

You may
already
know

Base on balls baseball rule on walking bases on errors, **Dysbasia** difficulty walking

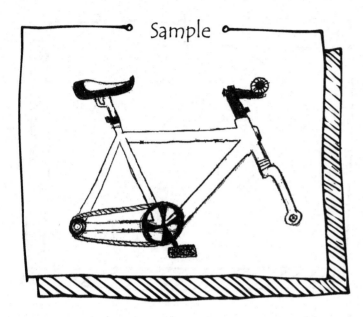

Sample

Consider a doodle of
a bicycle

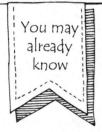

You may
already
know

Bicycle two-wheeled self-pedal machine, **Binoculars** using both eyes to look,
Bilateral affecting both sides, **Biaural** both ears

- 40 -

Consider a doodle of
a book

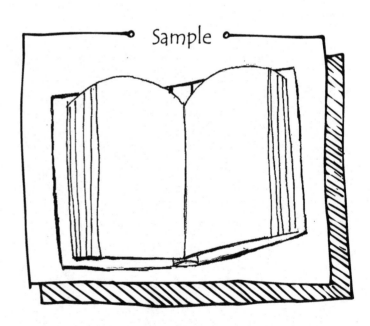

Sample

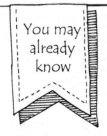

You may
already
know

Bibliography a list of books, **Bibliotherapy** use of books and reading as therapy

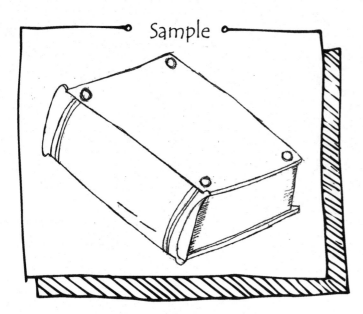

Sample

Consider a doodle of
a big book about
someone's life

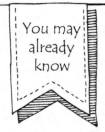

You may
already
know

Biology the science of life, **Biodegradable** breaks down with bacteria,
Biogenesis origin of life, **Biokinetics** science of movement of organisms

Consider a doodle of
happy new cells blasting
off

Sample

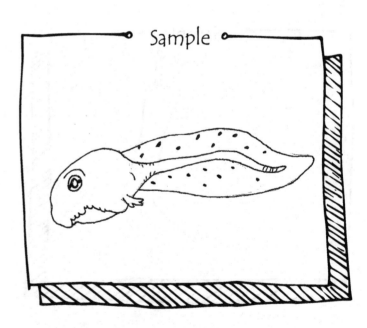

Blastomycosis any infection from yeast

- -

Consider a doodle of
an arm tattoo

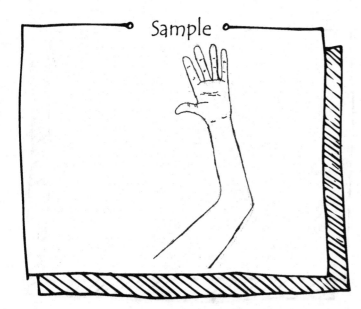

Sample

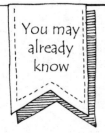

You may
already
know

Brachial pertaining to the arm, **Brachium** the arm from shoulder to fingers

Consider a doodle of
a short dog begging for
a bone

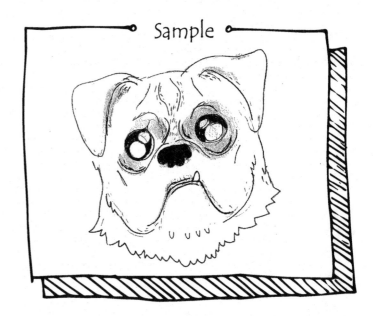

Sample

You may
already
know

Brachybasia shuffling, short step, **Brachydactyly** abnormally short fingers
and toes

Consider a doodle of
a turtle moving slowly

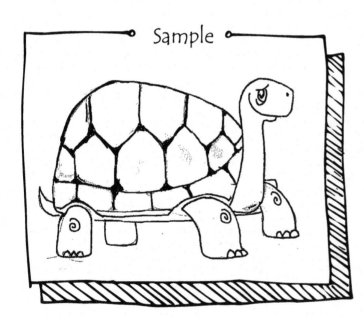

Sample

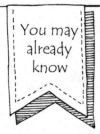

Bradykinesia abnormal slowness in movement, **Bradyesthesia** dull perception,
Bradycardia heart rate under 60 beats per minute, **Bradylalia** abnormally slow
speech

Consider a doodle of
a purse inflaming the
shoulder

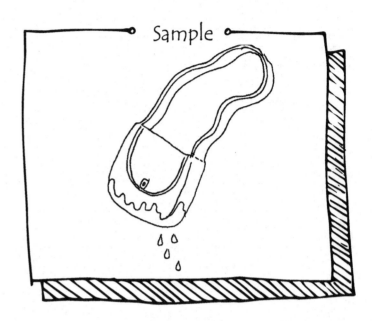

Sample

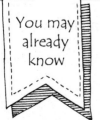

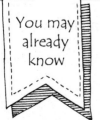
You may
already
know

Bursitis condition of inflammation the bursa, **Bursa** any fluid filled sac where friction occurs, **Bursolith** calculus in the bursa

Consider a doodle of
burning calories

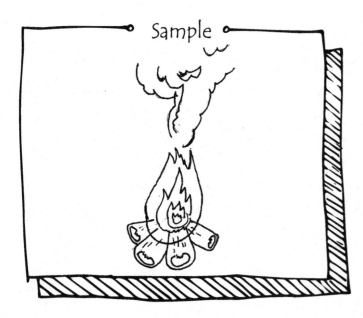

Sample

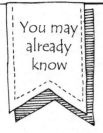
Calorie unit of heat required to burn its energy, **Calorific** producing heat,
Caloripuncture puncture using heat

Consider a doodle of
an ugly growth

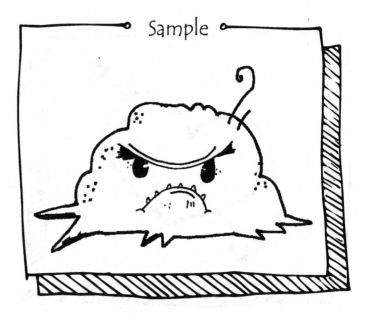

Sample

You may
already
know

Carcinogen causes cancer, **Carcinoma** malignant growth, **Carcinolysis** destruction
of cancer cells

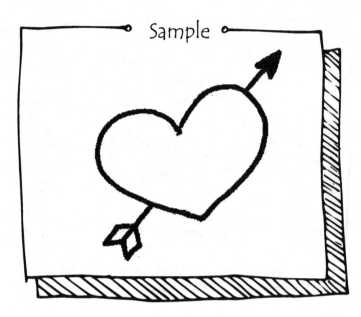

Sample

Consider a doodle of
a heart with artery letters:
C, A, R, D, I

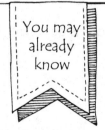

Cardiology concerned with heart health, **Cardiomyopathy** heart disease,
Cardiac cirrhosis liver disease complicating heart health, **Cardiotherapy** treatment
of heart disease

Consider a doodle of
bracelets

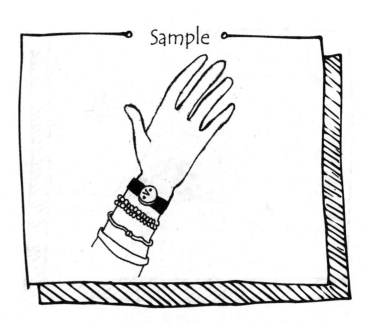

Sample

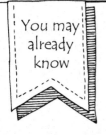

You may
already
know

Carpoptosis wrist drop, **Carpophalangeal** pertaining to the hand,
Carpitis inflammation of the synovial membranes of the hand

Consider a doodle of
underground letters:
C, A, T, A

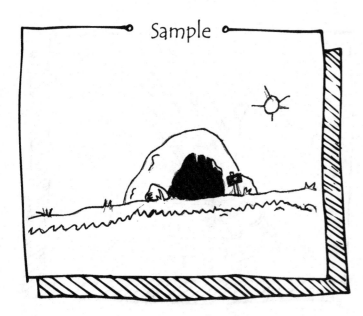

Sample

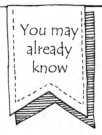

You may already know

Catatonic in a stupor and unable to move, **Catathymic** psychiatric conditions with perseveration, **Catatropia** downward eye gaze

Consider a doodle of
cleaning agents

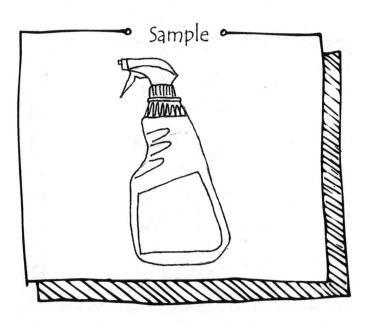

Sample

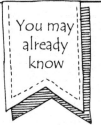

You may
already
know

Catharsis to bring to light something unconscious; an act of purging,
Cathartic drug cleaning agent for the bowels

- 53 -

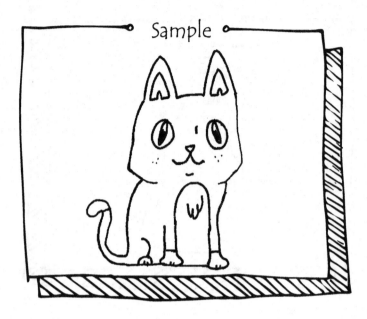

Sample

Consider a doodle of
a cat sitting on everything
in your house

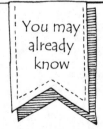

You may
already
know

Akathisia condition of marked motor restlessness and anxiety

Consider a doodle of
a cave

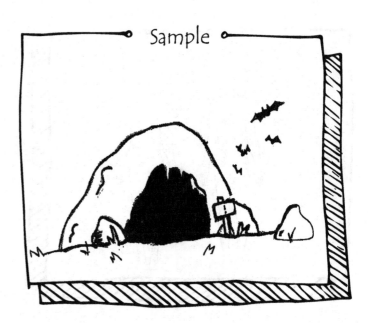

Sample

Cave hole in the earth, **Cavity** hole in a tooth, **Cavernostomy** surgery to drain a pulmonary abscess

Consider a doodle of
balloons

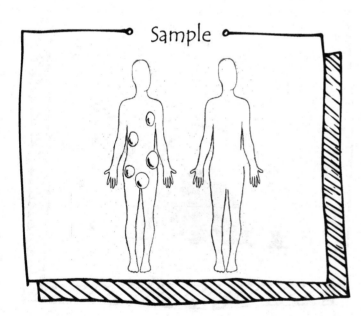

Sample

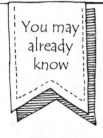

You may
already
know

Enterocele intestinal hernia, **Dermatocele** genetic skin condition of folds,
Craniocele brain protrusion of skull, **Enterocystocele** herniated bladder and
intestine

Consider a doodle of
a kangaroo with a pouch
on its abdomen

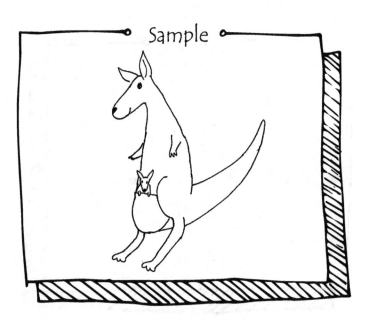
Sample

Celiac disease wheat or gluten digestion issues in the abdomen, **Celiac** pertaining
to abdomen, **Celitis** any abdominal inflammation

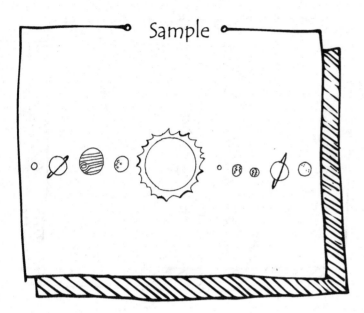

Sample

Consider a doodle of
anything in a center

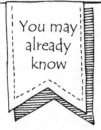
Central pertaining to the middle, **Centromere** constricted portion of
chromosome

Consider a doodle of
letters inside a brain:
C, E, R, E, B, R

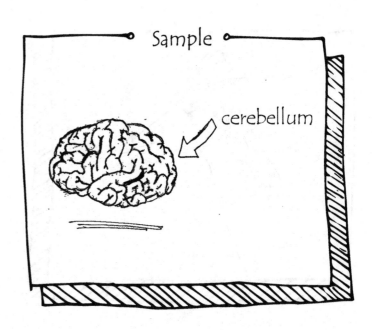

Sample

cerebellum

You may
already
know

Cerebellum part of the back of the brain, **Cerebropathy** any brain disease,
Cerebrospinal pertaining to the brain and spinal cord

Consider a doodle of
a giraffe with a long neck

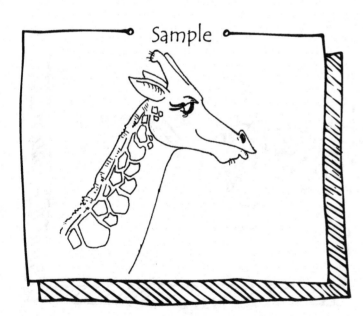

Sample

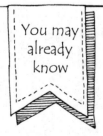

You may already know

Cervical pertaining to the cervix, **Cervicoplasty** plastic surgery of the neck, **Cervicobrachialgia** pain in the neck and arm due to pressed nerves

Consider a doodle of
chemicals boiling over

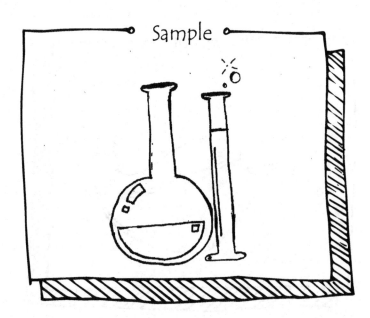

Sample

Chemotherapy chemical treatment of cancer, **Chemabrasion** superficial
destruction of the skin to prevent skin cancer or remove tattoos

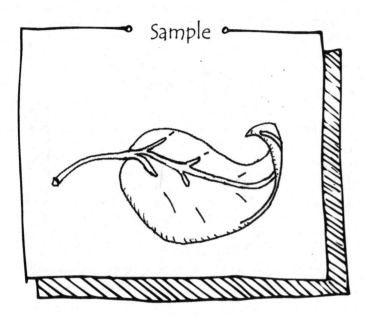

Sample

Consider a doodle of
a leaf shaped like the
letter C

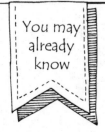

You may
already
know

Chloride makes plants green, **Chloruria** excess chlorides in urine,
Chlorophane green-yellow color in eyes

Consider a doodle of
sharks full of cartilage

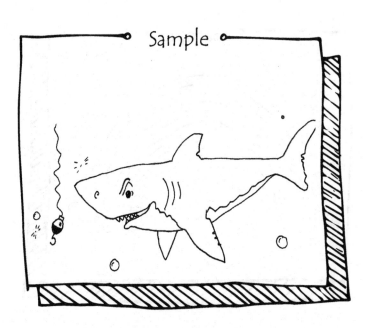

Sample

You may
already
know

Chondrosis formation of cartilage, **Chondroblastoma** benign tumor in epiphysis of bone, **Chondrodynia** pain in cartilage, **Chondromalacia** abnormal softening of the cartilage

Consider a doodle of
a colorful rainbow

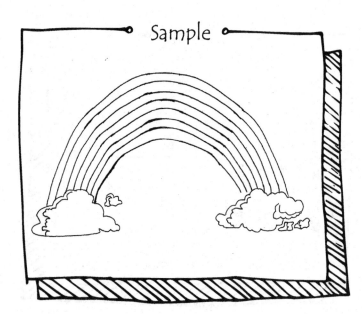

Sample

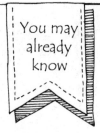

You may
already
know

Kodachrome color film used in cameras, **Chromosome** DNA visible with staining, **Chromophage** pigmentation, **Chromodacryorrhea** bloody tears

Consider a doodle of
the letter C with a curve
or a circle

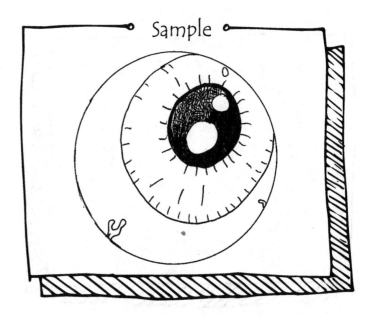

Sample

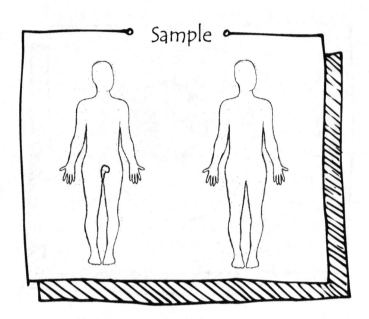

Sample

Consider a doodle of
a colon made out of
letters: C, O, L, O

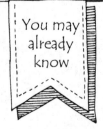

You may
already
know

Colonoscopy visual inspection of the colon, **Colopexy** surgical fixation of the
colon

Consider a doodle of
a universal warning sign

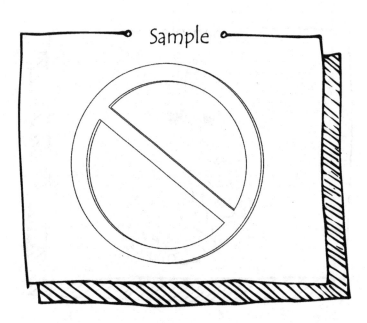

Sample

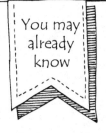

You may
already
know

Contraindicated against indications, **Contraception** prevention of pregnancy, **Contralateral** opposite side, **Contrecoup** injury on opposite side of brain from impact, **Contracture** shortening of muscle

Consider a doodle of
a bridge between the top
sections of the brain

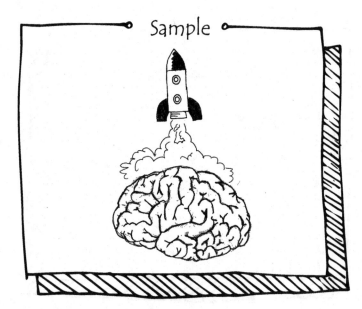
Sample

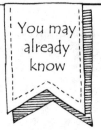
You may
already
know

Cortex top of the brain, **Corticobulbar** pertaining to cortex and medulla

Consider a doodle of
letters in ribs: C, O, S, T

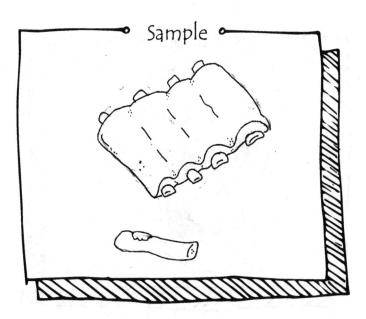

Sample

Costoclavicular pertaining to ribs and clavicle, **Costosternal** pertaining to ribs and sternum

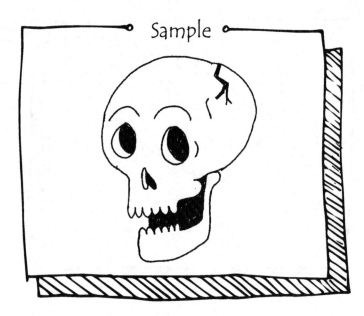

Sample

Consider a doodle of
a skull

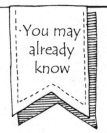

You may
already
know

Cranium (Hasbro) a game to test your knowledge, **Craniectomy** excision of a
brain segment, **Craniofacial** pertaining to skull and face

Consider a doodle of
a sign in the snowman's
hands saying CRYO

Sample

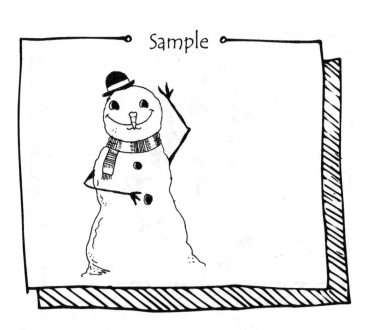

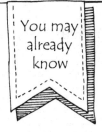

Cryogenic producing low temperature, **Cryotherapy** treatment with cold, **Cryometer** thermometer for very cold temperatures, **Cryobank** facility for freezing and storing semen at a low temperature

Consider a doodle of
a bluebird

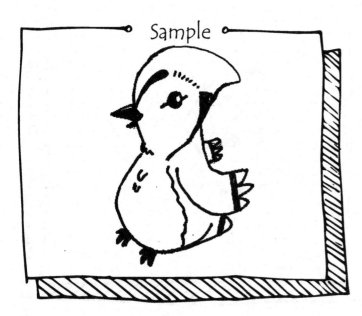

Sample

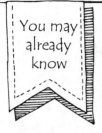
You may
already
know

Cyanosis blueish skin color, **Cyanopsia** vision with blue tinges, **Cyanogen** very poisonous gas that cuts off breathing

Consider a doodle of a
fluid-filled bladder

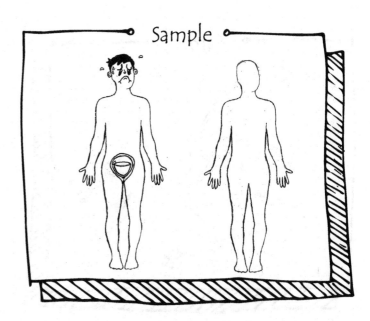

Sample

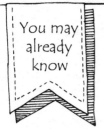

Cyst closed sac, **Cystectomy** removal of a cyst, **Microcyst** small cyst

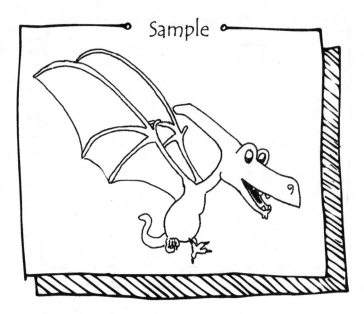

Sample

Consider a doodle of
flying dinosaurs

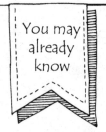

You may
already
know

Dactylography study of fingerprints, **Dactylogryposis** permanent flexion of
fingers, **Dactylology** communication by sign language

Consider a doodle of
critters with teeth

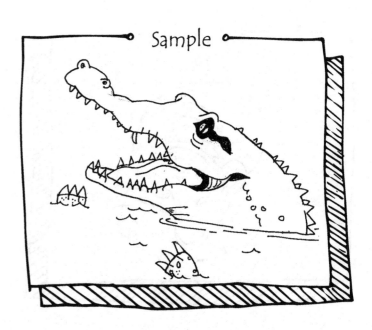

Sample

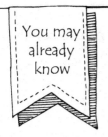

Dentist specializes in oral health, **Dentures** artificial teeth

Consider a doodle of
letters on skin:
D, E, R, M, O

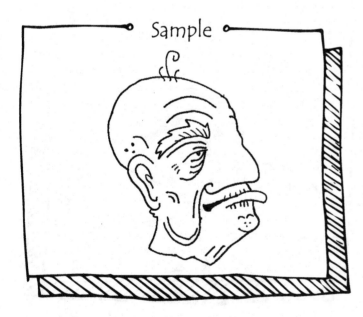

Sample

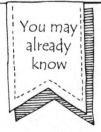

You may
already
know

Dermatologist specializes in skin health, **Dermoid** skin cyst, **Dermatosis** condition
of the skin, **Dermatoheteroplasty** skin graft from another species

Consider a doodle of
two of anything

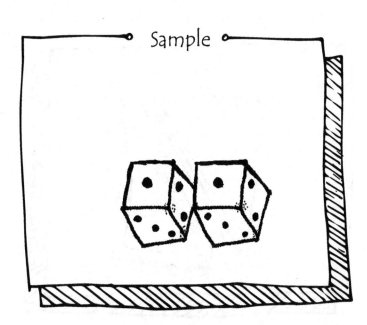

Sample

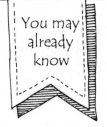
Dice two or more die, **Didactylous** only two digits on hand or feet

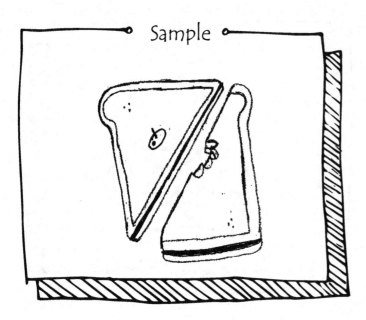

Sample

Consider a doodle of
sandwiches cut on the
diagonal

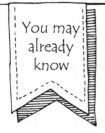
Dialysis artificial removal of waste from the blood, **Diagnosis** through evaluation, **Diabrotic** ulcerated through, **Director** grooved instrument to guide a surgical instrument

Consider a doodle of
double dip ice cream

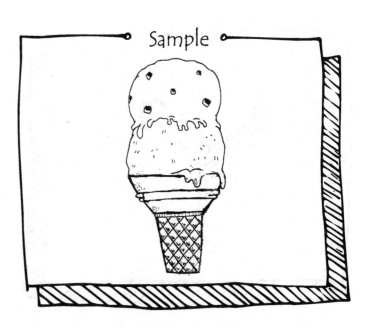

Sample

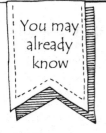

You may
already
know

Diplopia double vision, **Diploid** two sets of chromosomes,
Diplomyelia lengthwise fusion of spinal cord appearing as two cords

Consider a doodle of
fancy drinks

Sample

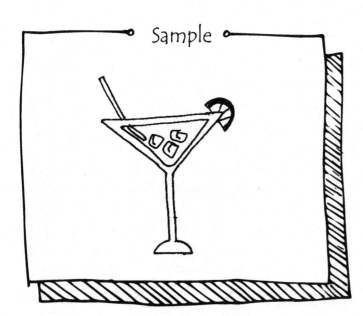

You may
already
know

Dipstick measures liquid in cars, **Dipsosis** excess thirst, **Dipsotherapy** therapeutic
limitation of fluids

Consider a doodle of
tubing in letters: D, I, S

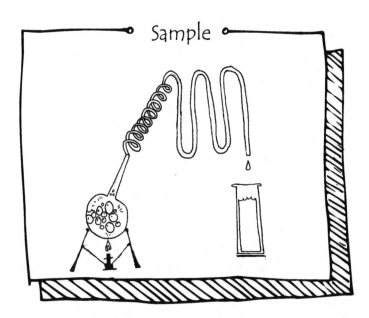

Sample

Consider a doodle of
far away communication

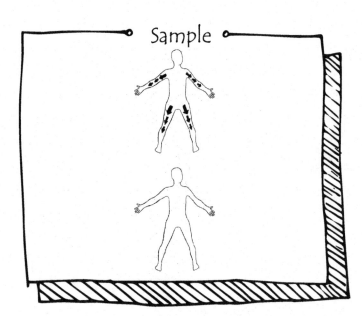

Sample

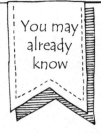

You may
already
know

Distribute to spread out, **Distal** away from the center, as in distal phalanges,
Distogingival distal wall of a tooth cavity

Consider a doodle of
two things running

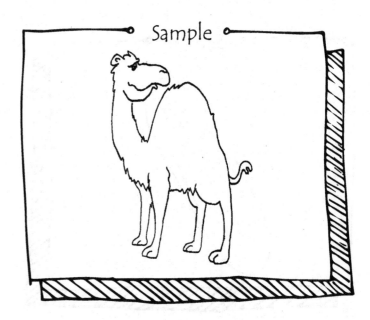

Sample

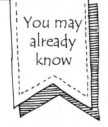
Dromedary camel running in the desert, **Syndrome** symptoms running together

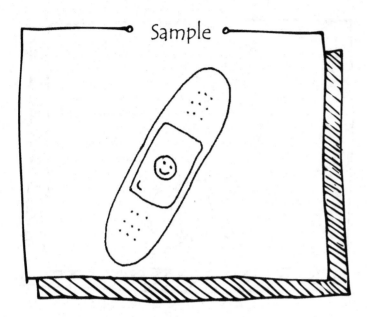

Sample

Consider a doodle of
a bandage

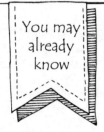

You may
already
know

Pododynia nerve pain in the heel of the foot, **Oneirodynia** nightmare,
Enterodynia intestinal pain

Consider a doodle of
messed up letters: D, Y, S

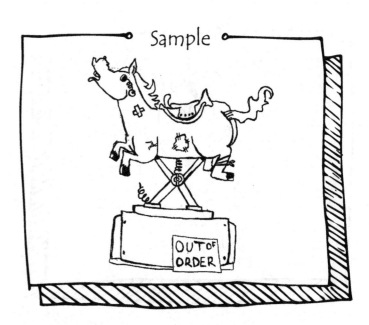

Sample

OUT OF
ORDER

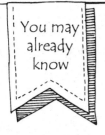

You may
already
know

Dysfunctional not functional, **Dystrophy** faulty nutrition, **Dyspnea** labored breathing, **Dyspepsia** indigestion, **Dyslexia** difficulty in reading, spelling, and writing

Consider a doodle of
ghostly letters: E, C, T, O

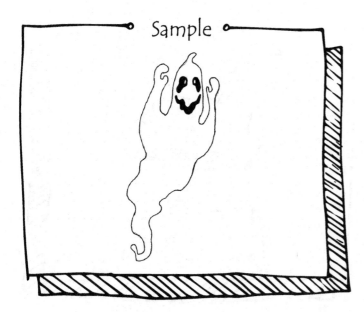

Sample

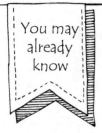

Tonsillectomy removal of the tonsils, **Hysterectomy** surgical removal of uterus
or surrounding parts, **Cryohypophysectomy** destruction of pituitary gland by
applying cold

Consider a doodle of
swollen letters:
E, D, E, M, A

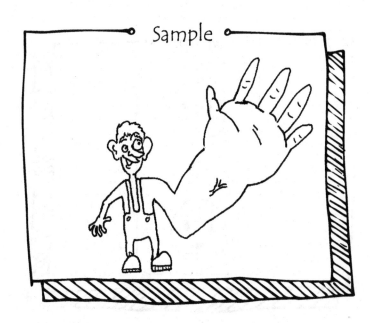

Sample

Edema swollen, **Cardiac edema** also known as congestive heart failure,
Edematogenic causing edema, **Pitting edema** when pressure leaves an
indentation

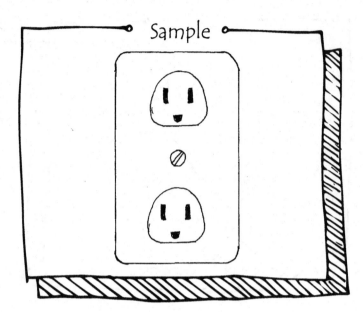

Consider a doodle of
electrical boxes

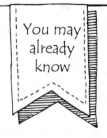

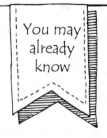 You may already know

Electrical pertaining to electricity, **Myoelectric** pertaining to the electric activity of a muscle, **Electroshock** applying electricity to the brain, **Electrostimulation** electrical treatment of tissues and muscles

Consider a doodle of
a vampire

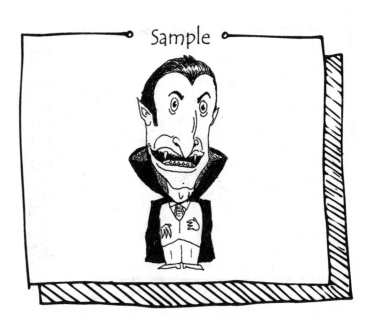

Sample

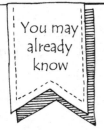

Anemia tired blood; abnormal red blood cells, **Leukemia** condition of white
blood cells

Consider a doodle of
bugs in stones

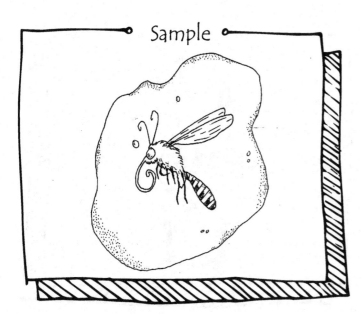

Sample

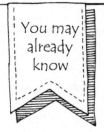

You may
already
know

Endocardial within the heart, **Endometriosis** abnormal tissue of the uterus,
Endocarditis inflammation of the lining of the heart, **Endocrine** inside the glands

Consider a doodle of
large brains

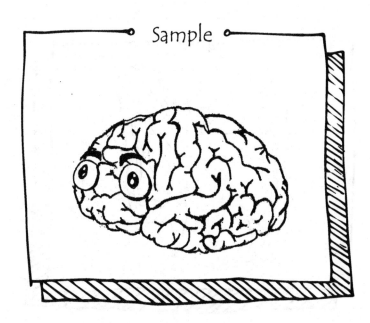

Sample

Encephalitis inflammation of brain, **Encephalomyelitis** inflammation of the brain
and spinal cord

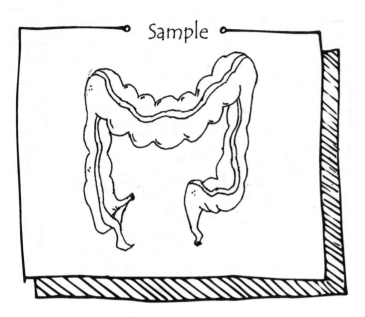

Sample

Consider a doodle of
the stomach emptying
into the intestines

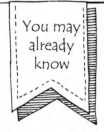

You may
already
know

Enteric-coated medicine medicine coated to prevent absorption until after reaching the stomach, **Enteroenterostomy** surgical joining of two parts of the intestines, **Enterorrhagia** hemorrhage of the intestines

Consider a doodle of
the top of the skin

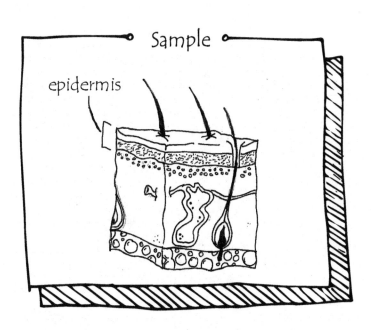

Sample

epidermis

You may
already
know

EpiPen (epinephrine) needle that pierces the skin to give medication,
Epidemic widely diffused and rapidly spreading, **Epicondyle** an eminence upon a
bone

Sample

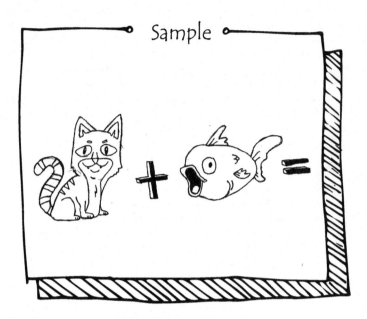

Consider a doodle of
two things that equal
something else

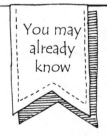

You may
already
know

Equilateral all sides equal, **Equilibrium** balance between two states,
Equiaxial equal axis length

Consider a doodle of
red fruit

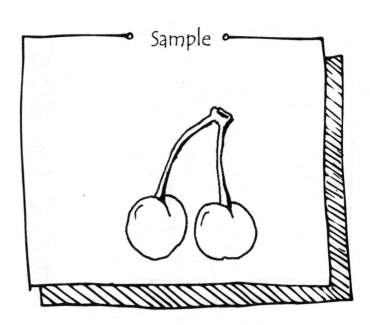

Sample

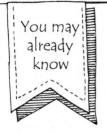

You may
already
know

Erythema abnormal red skin; sunburn, **Erythromycin** medication for
positive bacteria rods, **Erythremia** abnormal amount of red blood cells,
Erythrocyanosis mottled blueish-red discoloration of the legs when exposed
to cold

Consider a doodle of
a thumbs up

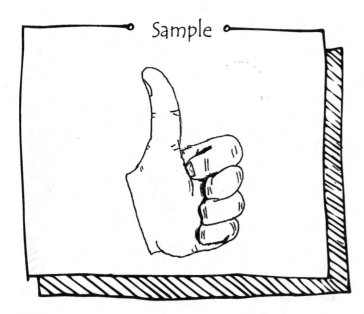

Sample

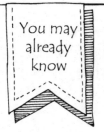

Eulogy speech about the positives of a person, **Euphoric** above normal happiness

Consider a doodle of
island rescues

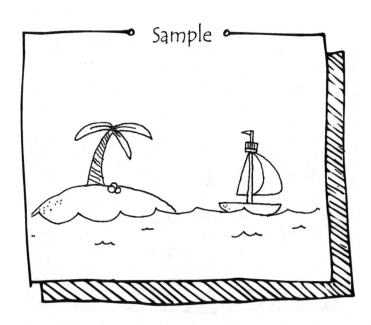

Sample

You may
already
know

Exhibit outwardly show, as signs or symptoms, **Exhale** to breath out, **Exert** to bring to action, **Exfoliation** falling off of scales or layers, **Expiration** termination or death

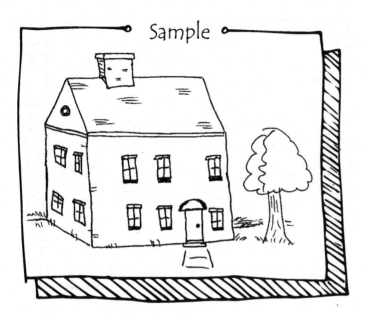

Sample

Consider a doodle of
the outside of anything

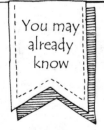
Exonerate free, **Exorcise** to get out an evil spirit, **Exocardia** outside wall of the
heart, **Exogenous** originate outside the source

Consider a doodle of
an extraterrestrial being

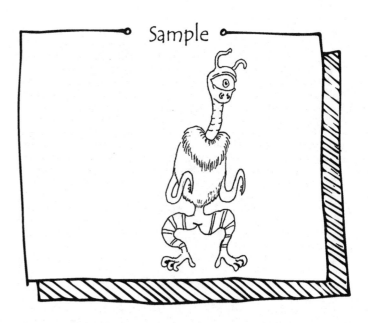

Sample

You may
already
know

Extract to draw out, **Extracurricular** activities outside the classroom,
Extraction process of pulling out, **Extramarginal** outside the limit of
consciousness

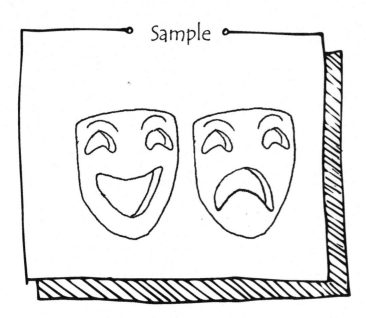

Sample

Consider a doodle of
faces

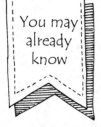

You may
already
know

Facial face treatment, **Faciolingual** pertaining to the face and tongue

Consider a doodle of
rope

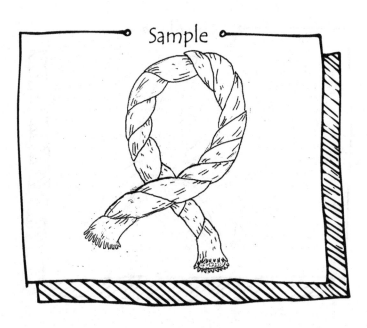

Sample

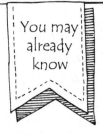

You may
already
know

Fiber grain, like a high-fiber bread, **Fibrosis** fibrous tissue

Consider a doodle of
candy

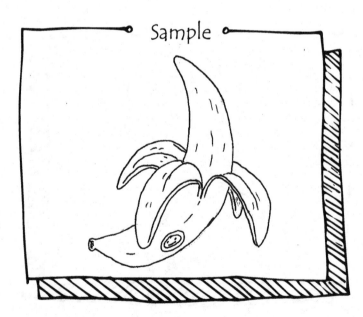

Sample

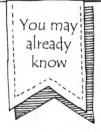

You may
already
know

Riboflavin yellow pigment widely seen in plants and animals, **Flavivirus** also
known as yellow fever

Consider a doodle of
straws

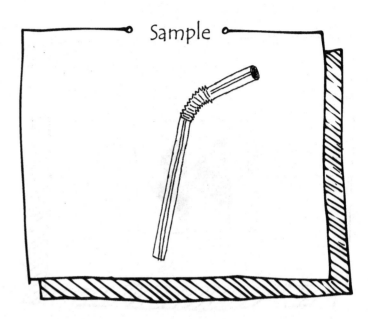

Sample

You may
already
know

Flexible capable of moving or changing, **Flexion** act of bending, **Flexor** a muscle
that flexes

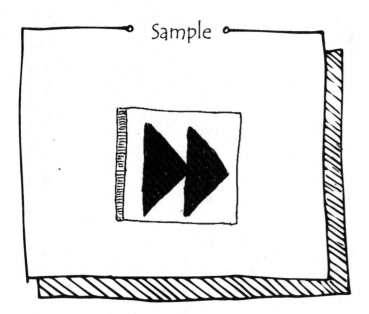

Sample

Consider a doodle of
a forward DVD button

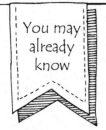

You may
already
know

Forerunner one that leads, **Foresight** power to see the future, **Forearm** part of
the arm before the wrist, **Forehead** before the eyes

Consider a doodle of
a functional machine

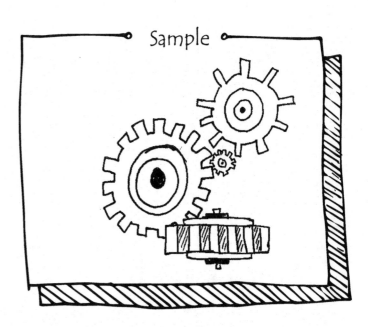

Sample

| You may already know | **Function** perform well; in balance, **Functional** affects the function but not the structure |

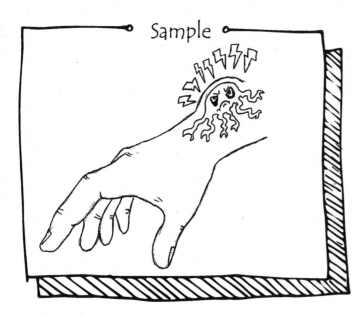

Sample

Consider a doodle of
screaming nerves

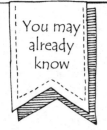

You may
already
know

Ganglion mass of tangled nerve cells outside the central nervous system,
Gangling awkwardly built, **Ganglionectomy** removal of a ganglion,
Ganglioneuroma benign neoplasm composed of fibers

Consider a doodle of
a stomach with gas in it

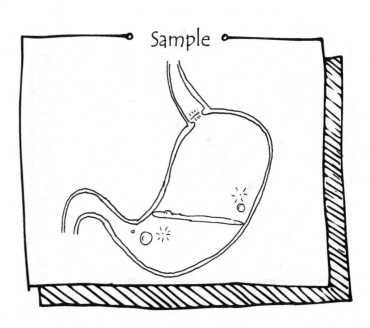
Sample

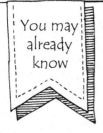

You may
already
know

Gastric juice stomach acid, **Gastronomy** art of eating good food,
Gastrointestinal pertaining to the stomach and intestines,
Gastrorrhagia hemorrhage in the stomach, **Gastrospasm** stomach spasms

Consider a doodle of
genes

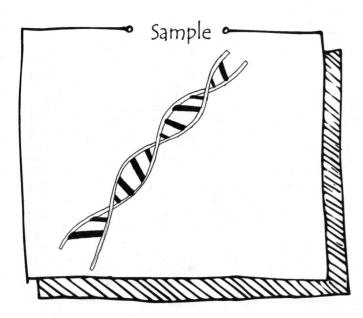

Sample

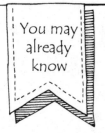

You may
already
know

Genealogy study of family history, **Paleogenetic** originating from the past,
Odontogenesis origin of teeth

Consider a doodle of
a honey bear

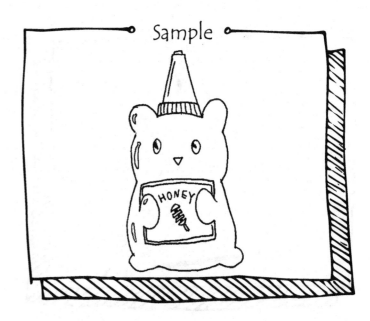

Sample

You may
already
know

Glucose sugar water, **Glycerin** sweet syrupy alcohol, **Hyperglycemia** high blood
sugar, **Glucosuria** sugar in urine

- 109 -

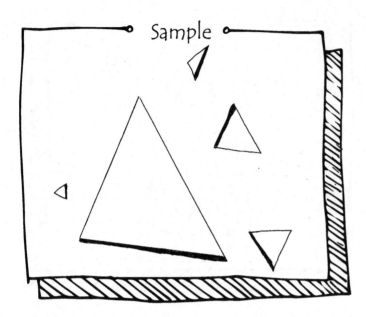

Consider a doodle of
triangles

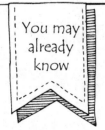

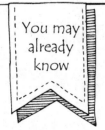
You may
already
know

Goniometer tool to measure angles, **Gonioscope** tool to look at the inside of
the eye

Consider a doodle of
a graduation cap

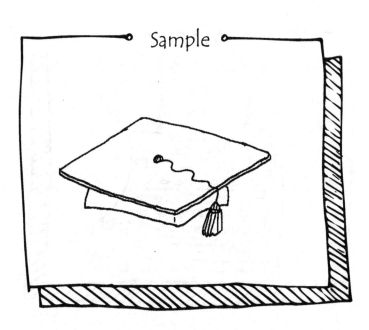

Sample

You may
already
know

Graduation successful steps, **Gradation** break down to steps, **Retrograde** step back
in history, **Gradient** rate of increase or decrease

Consider a doodle of handwriting like your Grandmother (Gram) writes

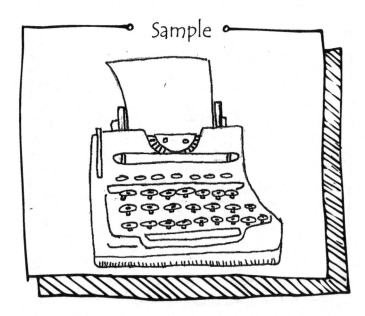

Sample

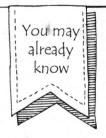

You may already know

Telegram written record delivered by wire, **Hepatogram** liver pulse by sphygmogram, **Phonocardiogram** record made of heart sounds

Consider a doodle of
a phonograph

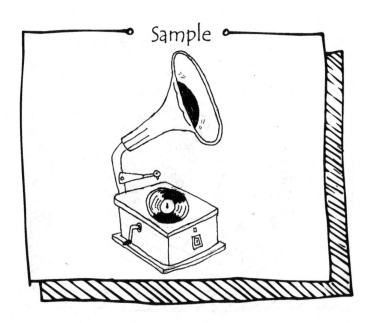

Sample

Phonograph used to play vinyl records, **Phonocardiograph** device for recording heart sounds, **Cryptolalia ographia** private written spoken language

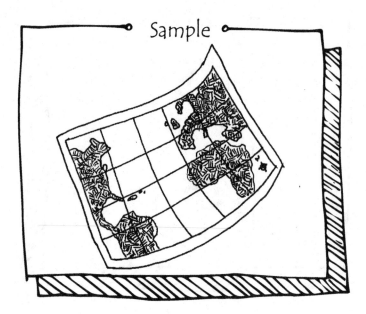

Sample

Consider a doodle of
a map

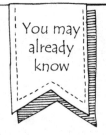
Photography captures photos, **Electromyography** the recording of electrical
activity of a muscle group

Consider a doodle of
a bag of blood

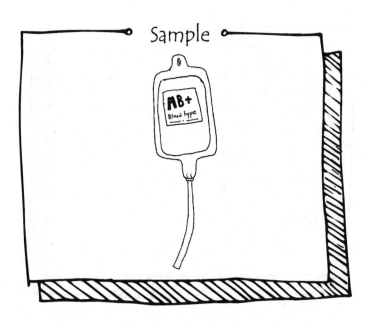

Sample

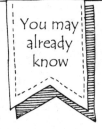

You may
already
know

Hemorrhage discharge of a large amount of blood, **Hemostat** holds blood vessel
closed as well as other uses, **Hemophilia** blood coagulation issues,
Hemopathy any blood disease

Consider a doodle of
half of something

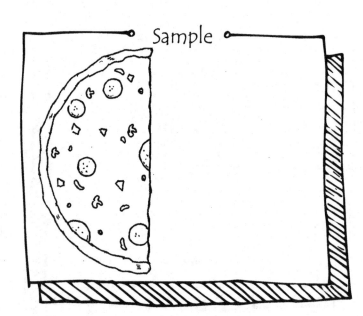

Sample

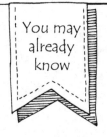

You may
already
know

Hemisphere half the earth, **Hemiplegia** paralysis on one side,
Hemiparaplegia paralysis on one side and lower half

Consider a doodle of
a liver

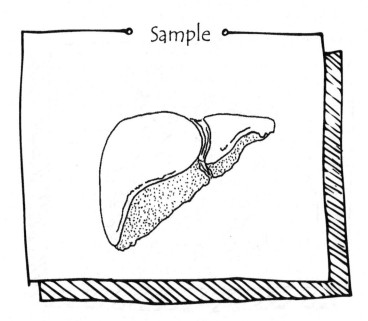

Sample

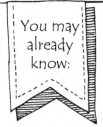

You may
already
know:

Heparin substance in liver that slows clotting, **Hepatomegaly** enlarged liver,
Hepatorrhexis ruptured liver

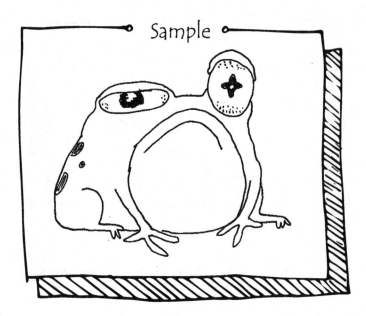

Sample

Consider a doodle of
a different-looking frog

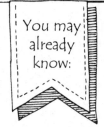

You may
already
know:

Heterosexual attracted to a different gender, **Heterotrichosis** growth of hair in
different colors

- 118 -

Consider a doodle of
twins

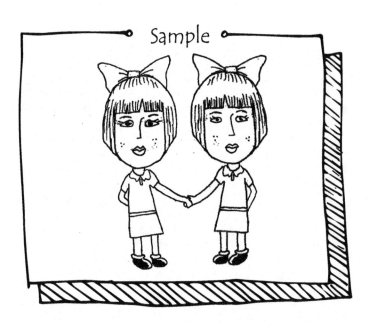

Sample

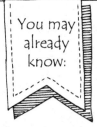

You may
already
know:

Homeostasis staying the same, **Homosexual** attracted to the same gender,
Homoplasis new tissue growth like the old

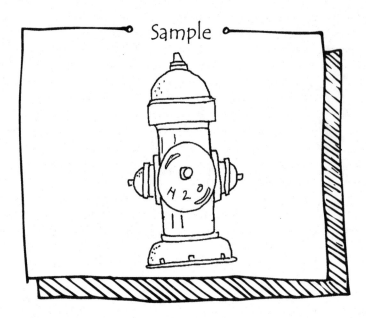

Sample

Consider a doodle of
a water hydrant

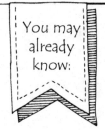
Hydrotherapy treatment in a pool, **Hydrokinetic** movement of water, as in a whirlpool

Consider a doodle of
a jumping puppy

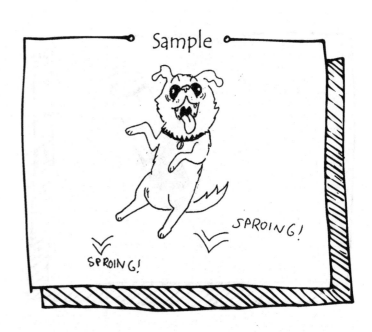

Sample

SPROING!

SPROING!

You may
already
know:

Hyperactive excessively active, **Hypertension** high blood pressure,
Hyperphagia increased appetite or intake

Consider a doodle of
a needle under the skin

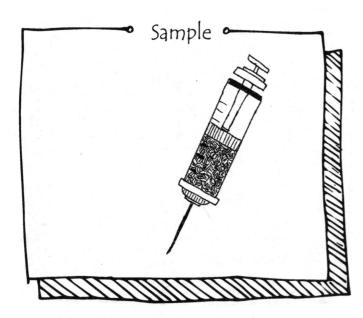

Sample

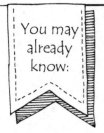
Hypnotist person who induces a sleep state, **Hypothyroidism** underactive thyroid
gland

Consider a doodle of degrees on the wall

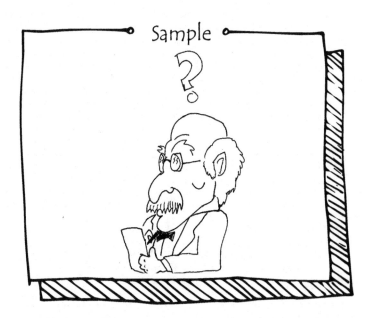

Sample

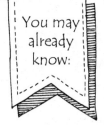

You may already know:

Psychiatrist mental health specialist, **Pediatrician** medical doctor for children

Consider a doodle of
a smart-looking person

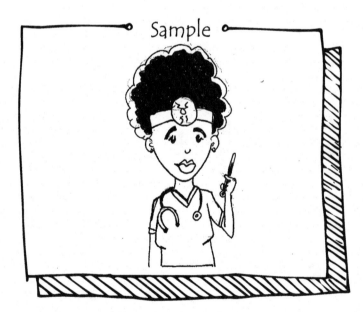

Sample

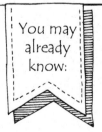

You may
already
know:

Physician medical doctor, **Esthetician** skin care specialist

Consider a doodle of
the internet

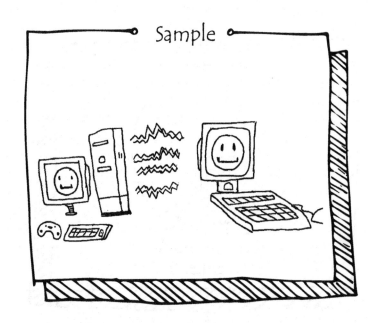

Sample

Interrupt breaking the continuity of something, **Intertwined** woven together,
Interoffice mail inside an organization, **Interface** boundary between systems,
Intervalvular between valves, **Intercostal** muscles in between the ribs

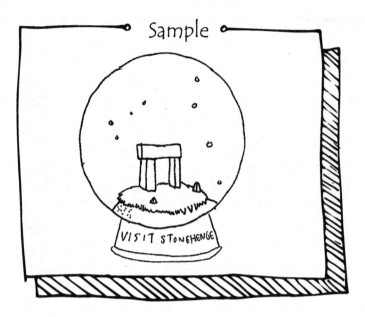

Sample

Consider a doodle of
a snow globe

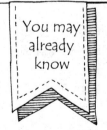**Intramural** sports within the walls of the college, **Intramuscular** within the muscle, **Intradermal** within the skin layers

Consider a doodle of
a professor

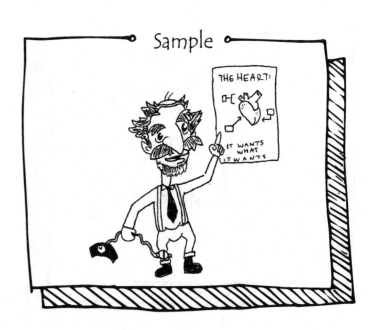

Sample

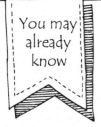

Cardiologist specializes in heart health, **Nephrologist** specializes in kidney health,
Physicist specializes in physics

Consider a doodle of
fireworks

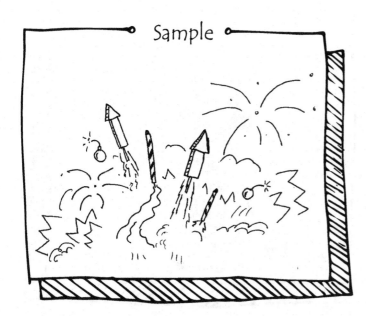

Sample

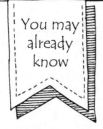

You may
already
know

Arthritis inflammation of the joints, **Hepatitis** inflammation of the liver

Consider a doodle of
a yellow banana

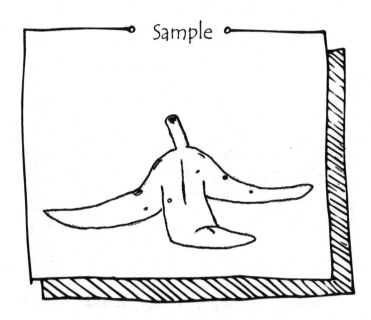

Sample

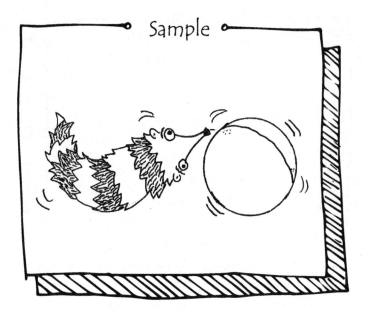

Sample

Consider a doodle of
moving toys

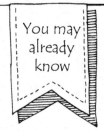
Kinetic sand toy that resembles sand and moves like water, **Kinesiology** study of movement, **Akathisia** motor restlessness

Consider a doodle of
a person arriving late on
the sidelines

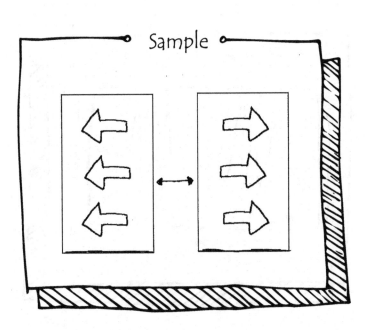

Sample

You may
already
know

Lateral away from the center; on the side, **Lateroduction** movement of a limb or eye to either side, **Lateral flexion** flexion on one side

Consider a doodle of
brain wave letters:
L, E, P, S, Y

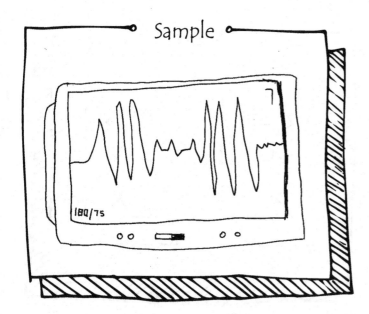

Sample

180/75

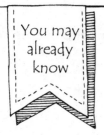

You may
already
know

Epilepsy seizure disorder, **Narcolepsy** sleep seizure

Consider a doodle of
something white

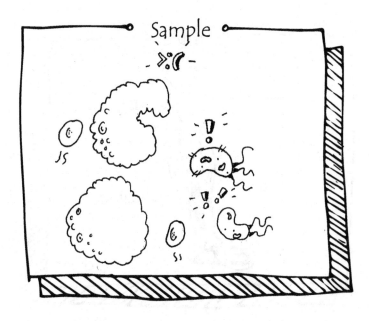

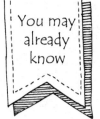

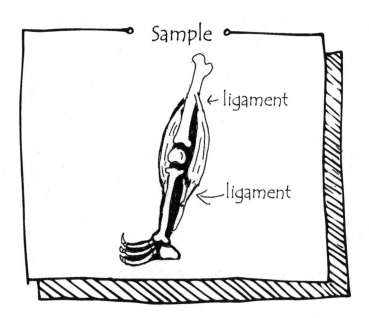

Sample

← ligament

← ligament

Consider a doodle of
connected letters:
L, I, G, A, M, E, N, T

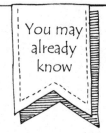

You may
already
know

Ligamentopexy fixation of the uterus by shortening the round ligament

Consider a doodle of
a fat cell

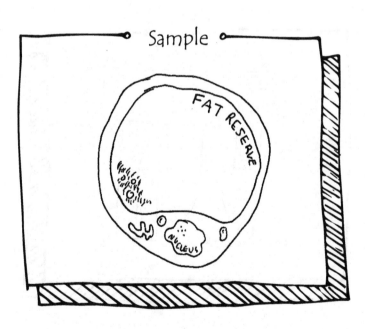

Sample

FAT RESERVE

NUCLEUS

Consider a doodle of
stone letters: L, I, T, H

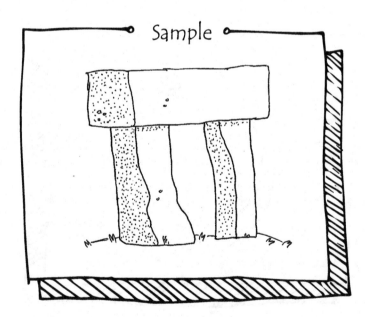
Sample

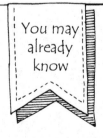
You may
already
know

Lithograph artistic print made from a flat, hard surface, such as stone,
Megalith large stone used in prehistoric monuments, **Tonsillolith** calculus in a
tonsil, **Lithotripsy** destruction of a kidney stone by ultrasonic waves

Consider a doodle that
uses letters in a speech
bubble: L, O, G

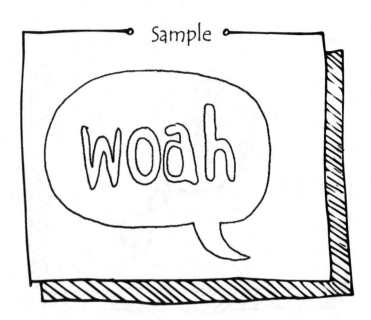

Sample

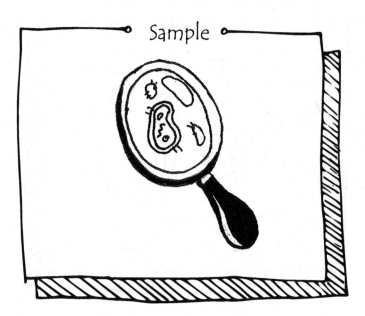

Sample

Consider a doodle of
a lens studying something

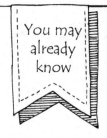

Cardiology study of heart health, **Nephrology** study of kidney health

Consider a doodle of
a pie chart

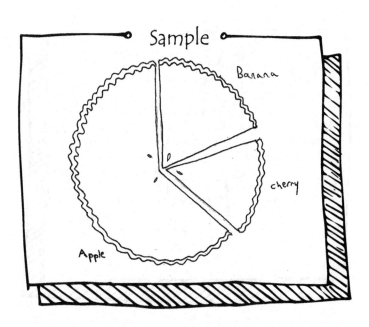

Sample

Banana

cherry

Apple

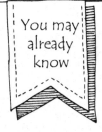

You may
already
know

Analysis exam by breaking into parts, **Odontolysis** resorption of dental tissue

Consider a doodle of
melting ice cream

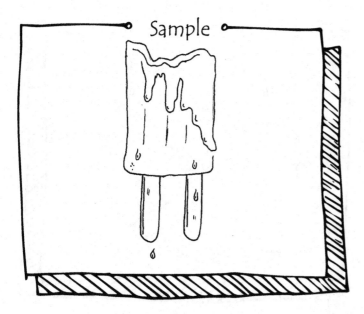

Sample

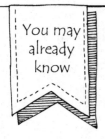

You may
already
know

Craniomalacia abnormal softening of the skull bones

Consider a doodle of
a mad scientist

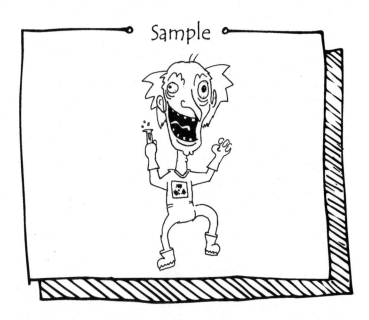

Sample

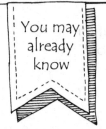

Mania excessive enthusiasm, **Maniacal** suggested of madness

Consider a doodle of
a medium stuffed bear in
a tree

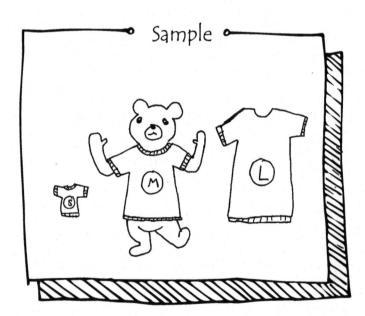

Sample

You may
already
know

Mediate act as intermediary, **Medius** situated in the middle, **Medium** person
communicating between the dead and living; average; middle position

Consider a doodle of
anything large

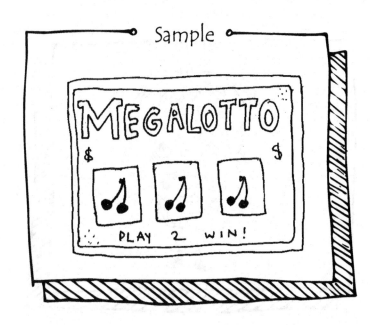

Sample

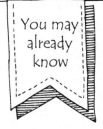

You may already know

Megaphone cone-shaped device to intensify sound, **Megabyte** millions of computer bytes, **Megavitamin** massive doses of vitamins, **Macrocosm** great world, **Macroscopic** visible to the naked eye

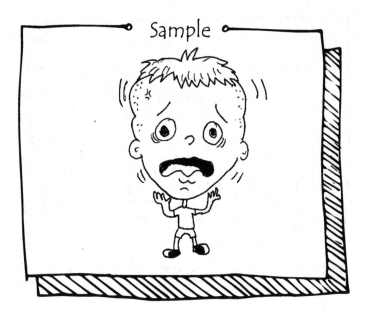

Sample

Consider a doodle of
a large-headed character

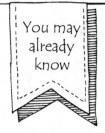

You may
already
know

Megalopolis very large city, **Megalomania** delusion of one's own extreme
greatness, **Megalodactyly** excessive size of fingers or toes

Consider a doodle of
spider legs

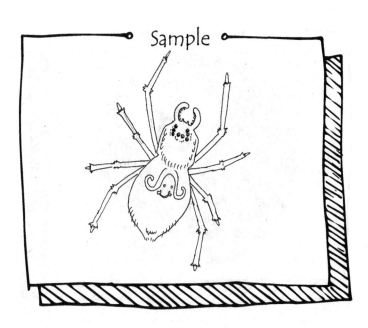

Sample

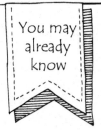

You may
already
know

Melodrama theatrical play with overacting and flailing limbs, **Melomelus** fetus
with impaired limbs, **Melodidymus** extra limbs

Consider a doodle of a
black billiard ball

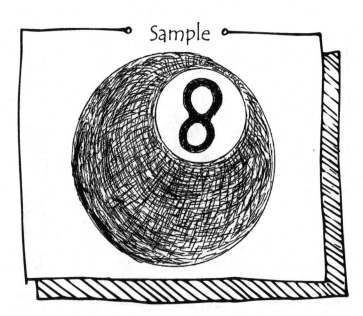

Sample

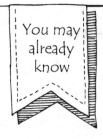

Melancholy depressed or gloomy spirits, **Melanoma** any tumor with black cells,
Melanism excessive pigment

Consider a doodle of
the middle of a donut

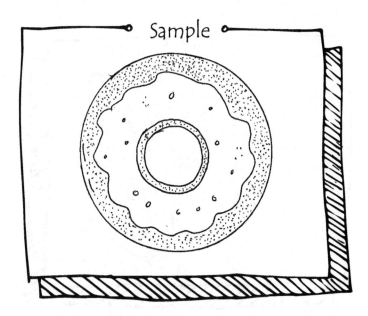

Sample

You may
already
know

Mesoderm middle layer of skin, **Mesosphere** sky between atmosphere and
thermosphere, **Mesocardia** atypical location of the heart

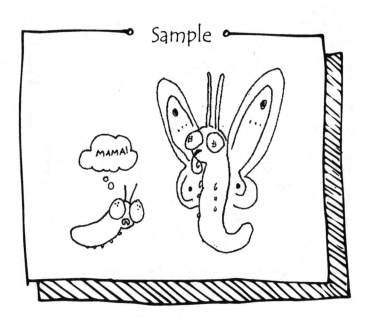

Consider a doodle of
butterflies after cocoons

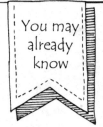

You may
already
know

Metacarpal bones of the hand that occur after the wrist, **Metabolism** sum of all
physical and chemical processes, **Meta-analysis** statistical process

Consider a doodle of
a meter

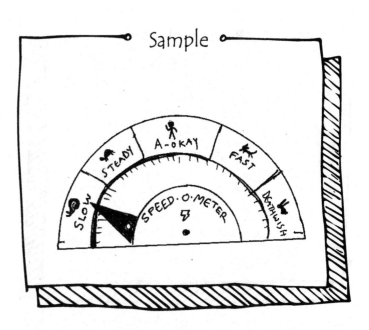

Sample

SPEED·O·METER

SLOW STEADY A-OKAY FAST DEATHWISH

You may
already
know

Thermometer measures temperature, **Sphygmomanometer** measures blood pressure, **Speedometer** measures the speed of a vehicle

Consider a doodle of
a ruler

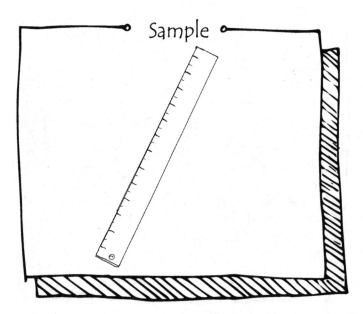

Sample

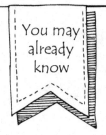

You may
already
know

Geometry math of measuring, **Phonometry** process of measuring sounds

micro-

one millionth (10^{-6}), small

Consider a doodle of
a microscope

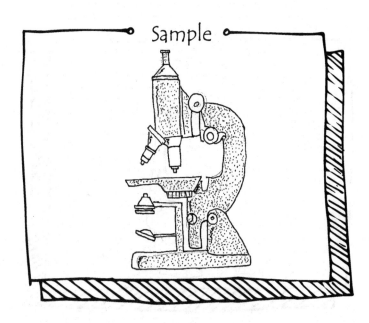

Sample

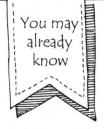

Microwave oven that cooks with small waves, **Microphone** device to transmit sound, **Microcephaly** abnormally small head, **Microsomia** abnormally small body, **Microsporosis** ring worm

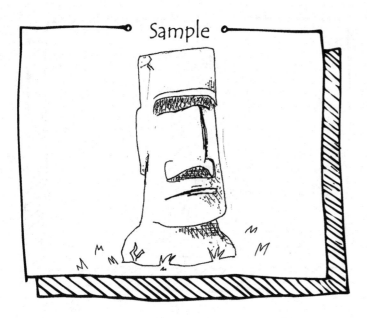

Sample

Consider a doodle of
a single mass of stones

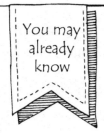

Mononucleosis blood disease common in young people,
Monobrachius one arm, **Monodactyly** presence of only one finger or toe,
Monomania preoccupation with one subject

Consider a doodle of
a multi-tool

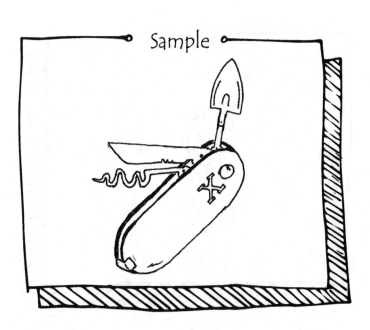

Sample

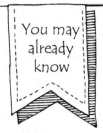

You may
already
know

Multiple many, **Multiarticular** affecting many joints, **Multiglandular** affecting
more than one gland

Consider a doodle of
a muscle man

Sample

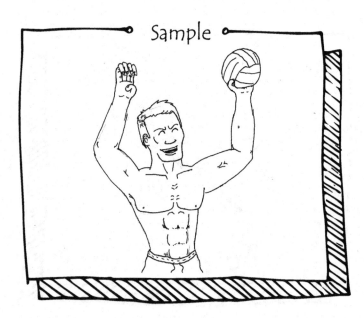

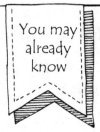
You may
already
know

Dermatomyositis collagen disease of skin and muscles with necrosis,
Myositis inflamed voluntary muscle, **Myofascial release** technique used to release
fascial tissue

Consider a doodle of
a spinal cord using letters:
M, Y, E, L

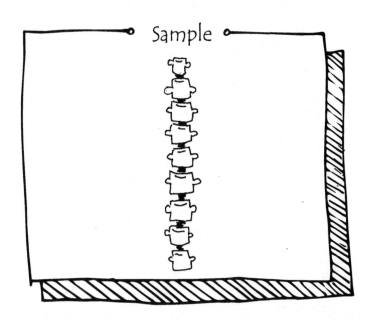

Sample

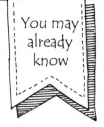

Myeloma tumor in bone marrow, **Myelin** fatty covering of nerves,
Myelocele herniated spinal cord, **Myelocyte** immature marrow cell or any gray
matter cell

Consider a doodle of
a sleepy kid

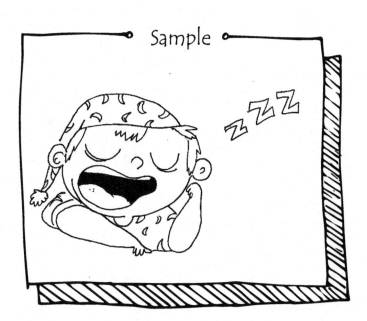

Sample

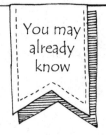

Narcotic controlled medicine due to addictions and stupor,
Narcolepsy uncontrolled sleep or stupor, **Narcohypnia** numbness felt on waking
from sleep

Consider a doodle of
a dead cell

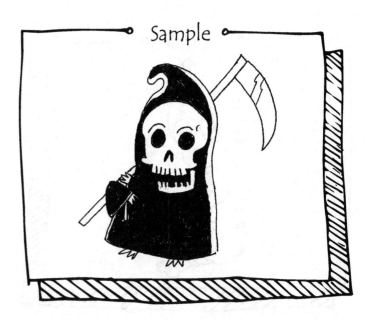

Sample

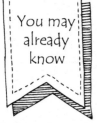

You may
already
know

Necrosis dead tissue, **Necrophilia** attraction to dead objects

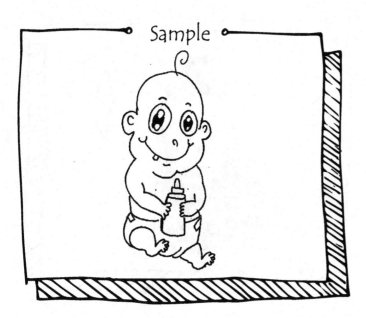

Sample

Consider a doodle of
a new baby

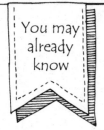

You may
already
know

Neoclassic adapting a classical style, **Neonate** newborn baby

Consider a doodle of
two kidneys

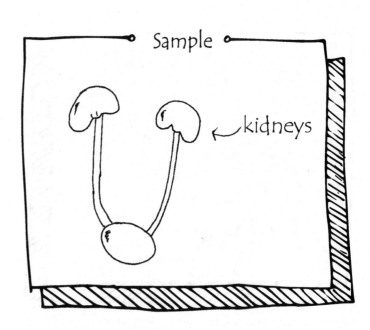

Sample

kidneys

Nephritis inflammation of the kidneys, **Nephrolith** kidney stone,
Nephropyelography radiograph study of the kidneys and pelvis

Consider a doodle of
a nerve

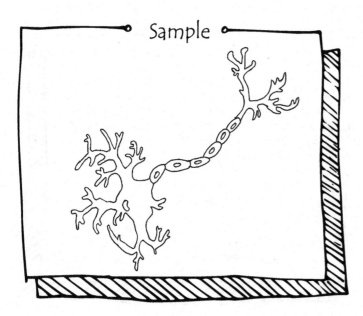

Sample

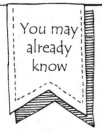

You may
already
know

Neuroscience study of the brain and nerves, **Neuron** cell of the nervous system

Consider a doodle of
an owl up all night

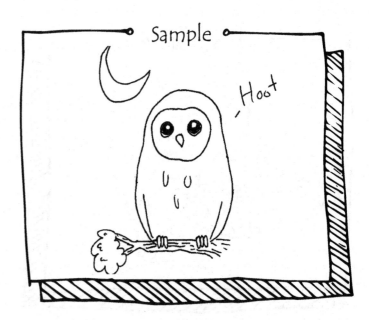

Sample

Hoot

You may
already
know

Nocturnal active at night, **Nocturia** excessive urination at night,
Noctiphobia fear of night

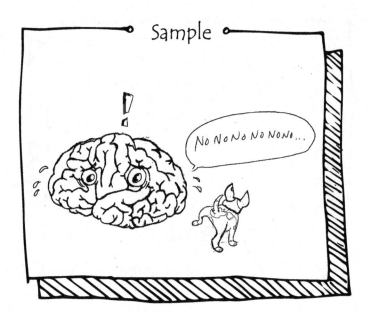

Consider a doodle of
a firm mind saying, "No!"

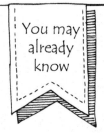

Paranoia mental illness characterized by delusions

Consider a doodle of
a box of cereal

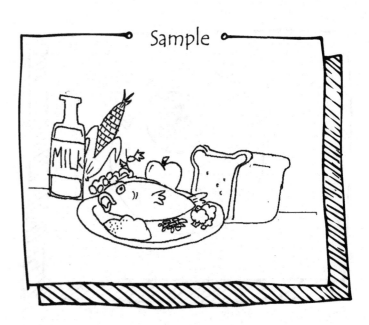

Sample

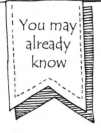 **Nutrition** act of nourishing, **Nutriture** status of body in nutrition,
Nutriment food

- -

Consider a doodle of
eyes in letters: O, C, U, L

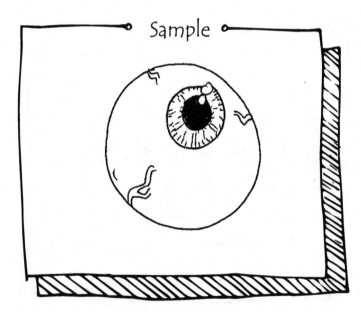

Sample

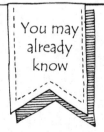

You may already know

Ocular lens eyepiece, **Oculomotor** affecting eye movements,
Oculocutaneous pertaining to the eye and the skin around it

Consider a doodle of
a toothy smile

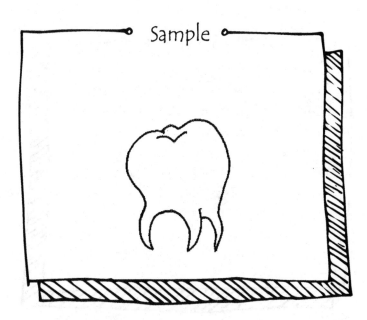

Sample

Odontopathy disease of teeth

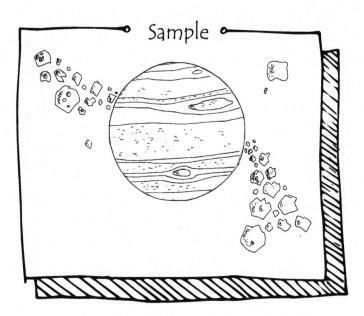

Sample

Consider a doodle of
other planets

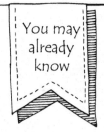**Fibroid** fiber-like mass, **Lipoid** resembling fat, **Paranoid** resembling paranoia,
Schizoid resembling schizophrenia

Consider a doodle of
slow work animals

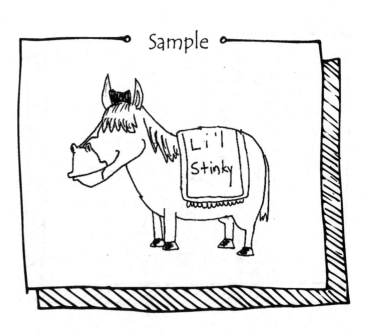

Sample

Consider a doodle of
flower letters:
O, L, F, A, C, T

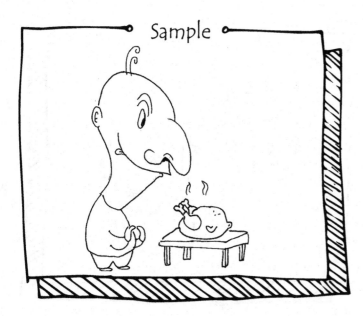

Sample

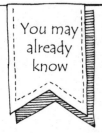

You may
already
know

Olfactology science of smell, **Olfactometer** instrument to test sense of smell

Consider a doodle of
a cancer cell

Sample

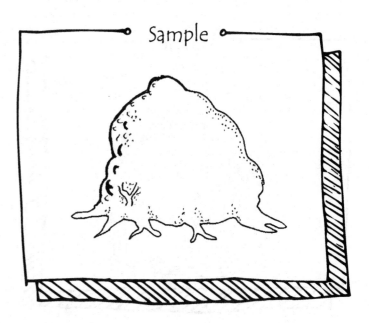

Lymphoma cancer of lymphoid tissues, **Sarcoma** tumor that starts in bone, cartilage, or muscle

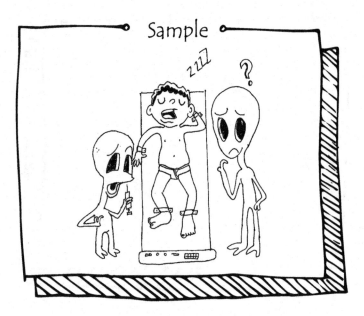

Sample

Consider a doodle of
an alien autopsy

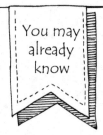
Autopsy exam after death

Consider a doodle of
braces

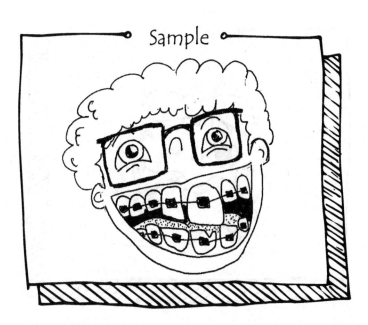

Sample

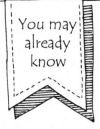
You may
already
know

Orthodontist dentist who uses braces to straighten teeth, **Orthotic** device to straighten, **Orthograde** walking upright

- -

Consider a doodle of
a sick person

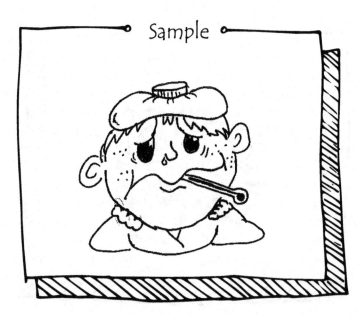

Sample

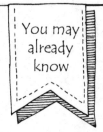

You may
already
know

Cyanosis condition of blue skin, **Otomycosis** fungal infection of the ear canal

Consider a doodle of
a happy dog with a bone

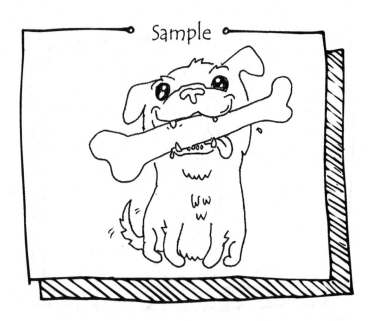

Sample

Osteoporosis frail bones, **Osteoarthritis** inflammation and degeneration of
joints, **Osteomyelitis** bacterial infection of a bone; more common in children

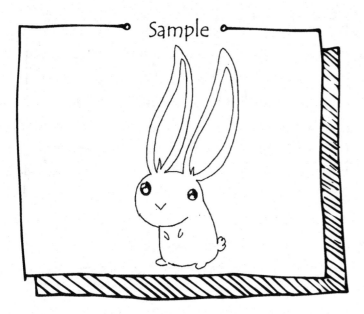

Sample

Consider a doodle of
a big-eared animal

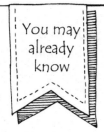**Otoscope** tool to look in an ear, **Otosclerosis** spongy bone in the labyrinth of
the ear, **Otoencephalitis** inflammation of the brain due to inflamed middle ear

Consider a doodle of
an elephant

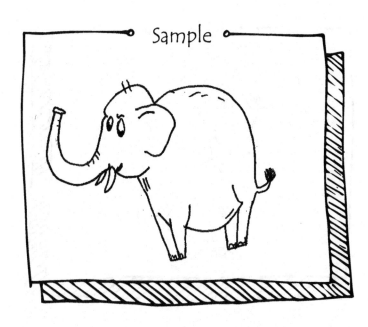

Sample

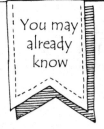

You may
already
know

Pachyderm an animal with thick skin, such as an elephant, **Pachydactyly** enlarged,
thick fingers or toes, **Pachyglossia** thick tongue, **Pachynsis** abnormal thickening

Consider a doodle of
a dinosaur bone

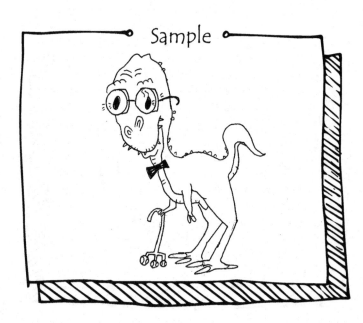

Sample

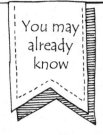

Paleo diet diet based on foods available during the Paleolithic era,
Paleocerebellum older parts of the brain, specifically those that address flow,
Paleopathology study of disease in bodies preserved from ancient times

Consider a doodle of
an ice pack

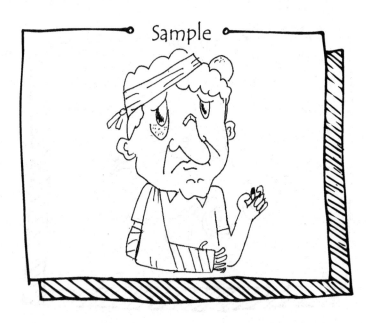

Sample

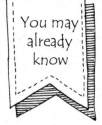

You may
already
know

Palliative affording relief, especially end of life, **Palliate** to relieve symptoms

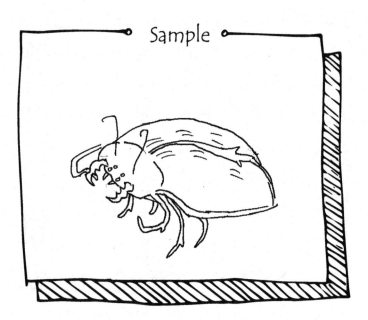

Sample

Consider a doodle of
a bug that lives near you

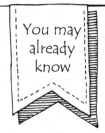
You may
already
know

Parapsychology beyond traditional psychology, **Parasite** organism that lives
on or along with a host, **Paraplegia** without movement of lower (tetraplegia)
extremities

Consider a doodle of
a walker for partial paralysis

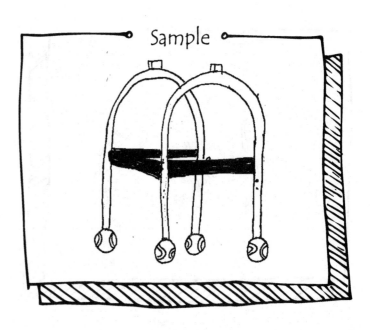

Sample

Hemiparesis weakness on one side of the body, **Paraparesis** partial paralysis of lower extremities, **Myoparesis** slight paralysis, **Monoparesis** weakness in a single part

Consider a doodle of
a fight to the death against
disease

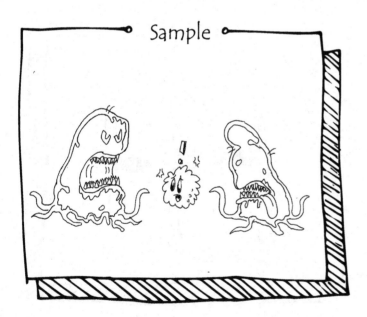

Sample

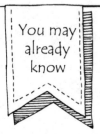
Pathology study of diseases, **Pathogenetic** disease causing, **Phonopathy** disease of organs of speech

Consider a doodle of
the pause button on a
DVD player

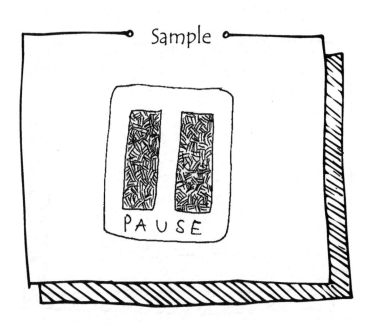

Sample

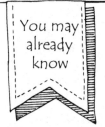

Menopause menstrual periods ending, **Diapause** state of inactivity

Sample

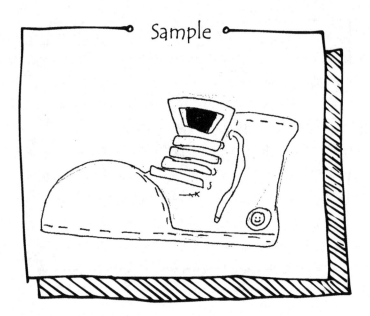

Consider a doodle of
a child's sneaker

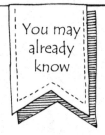

Pedicure foot treatment, **Pediatric** specializes in child's health,
Pedodontist dentist for children, **Pedodynamometer** instrument to measure
leg strength

Consider a doodle of
not enough money

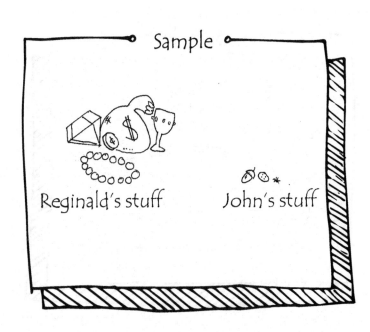

Sample

Reginald's stuff

John's stuff

Leukopenia deficiency in the number of white blood cells, **Orthopnea** difficulty breathing unless upright

Consider a doodle of
a submarine with a
periscope

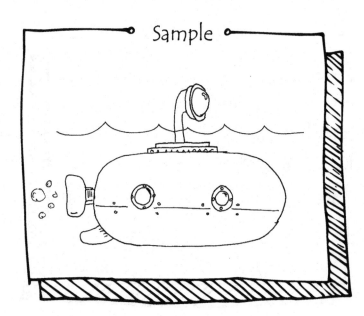

Sample

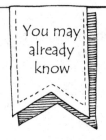

You may
already
know

Periscope instrument to see around blocked views, **Peritoneum** layer around an
organ, **Peripheral nervous system** nerves around the body

Consider a doodle of
Pexy brand glue

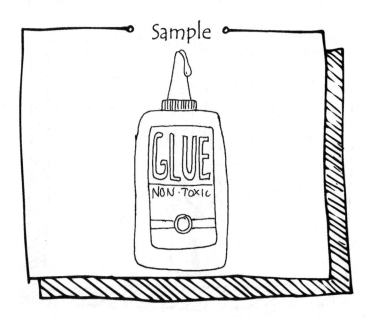

Sample

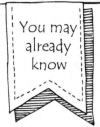

You may
already
know

Cystopexy bladder fixed to abdominal wall

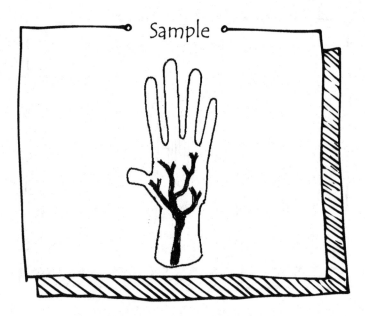

Sample

Consider a doodle of
veins in the hand

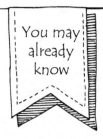

You may
already
know

Phlebotomy the process of puncturing or cutting into veins,
Phlebosclerosis thickening of vein walls

Consider a doodle of
a scary clown

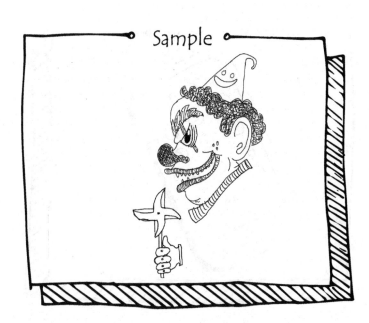

Sample

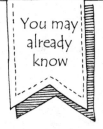

You may already know

Claustrophobia fear of small places, **Phonophobia** morbid dread of speaking out loud, **Panphobia** fear of everything

Consider a doodle of
a cell phone

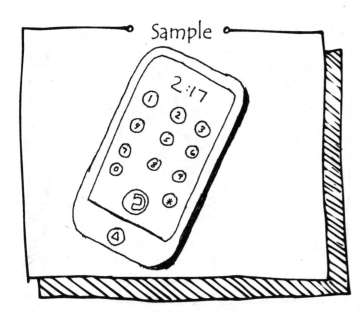

Sample

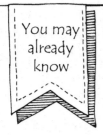
Phonograph machine that plays music, **Phonic** pertaining to voice,
Xylophone sound instrument of wood, **Phonometer** device to measure sound,
Phonomassage treatment of ear disease by musical vibration

Consider a doodle of
a camera

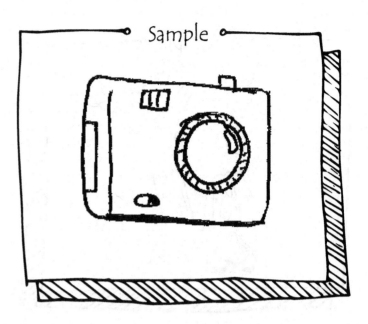

Sample

You may
already
know

Photograph picture from exposure to light, **Photocopy** reproduction of a
document using light, **Photosensitive** aversion to light, often due to a medical
issue or medication

- 189 -

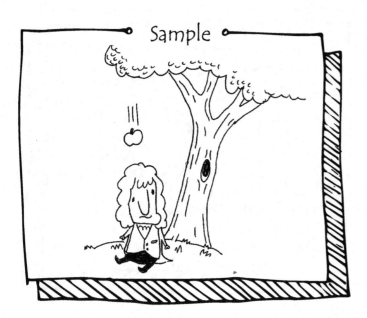

Sample

Consider a doodle of
an apple falling on Isaac
Newton's head

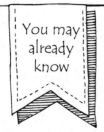
Physical therapy using physical methods in rehabilitation,
Physiopathologic pertaining to disease of cells, **Physiological** pertaining to cells

Consider a doodle of
growing letters:
P, H, Y, S, I, S

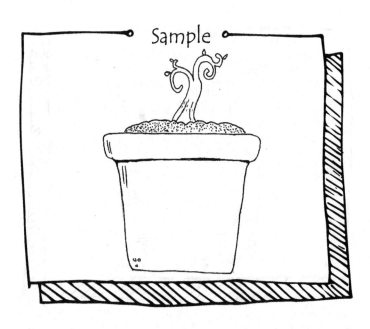

Sample

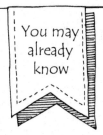

Epiphysis the growth center of long bones

Consider a doodle of
tools on a wall

Sample

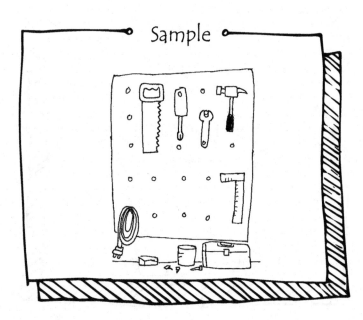

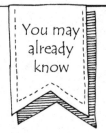

You may
already
know

Plastic surgery surgery to fix a cosmetic issue, **Cranioplasty** plastic surgery of
skull, **Dermatoplasty** plastic surgery on skin

Consider a doodle of
a handicap parking sign

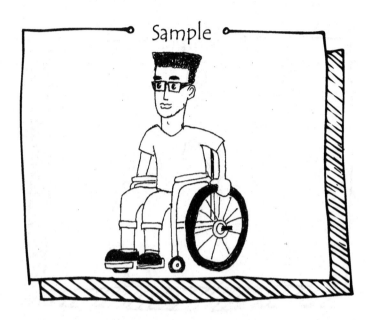

Sample

You may
already
know

Paraplegia paralyzed from the waist down, **Tetraplegia** or **quadriplegia** paralyzed
in four limbs

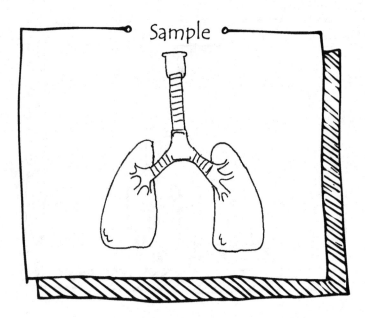

Sample

Consider a doodle of
lungs

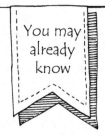

You may
already
know

Pneumonia condition of breathing, **Polypnea** hyper breathing

Consider a doodle of
footprints

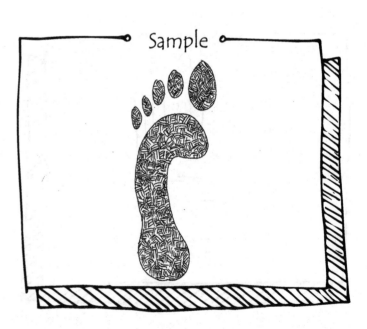

Sample

Podiatrist specializes in foot health, **Pododynamometer** measures footsteps,
Podarthritis inflammation of the foot joints

Consider a doodle of
a many-armed monster

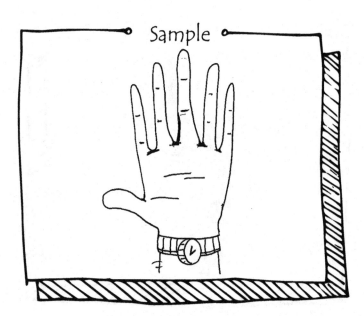

Sample

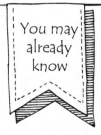

You may
already
know

Polygons shapes with many sides, **Polygamy** practice of having many spouses,
Polydactylism condition of over five digits on hands or feet,
Polydipsia excessive thirst, **Polyglandular** affecting many glands

Consider a doodle of
holey letters:
P, O, R, O, S, I, S

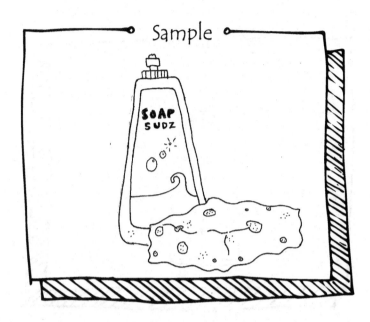

Sample

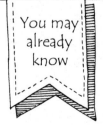
Osteoporosis thin bones, **Polyporus** having many pores

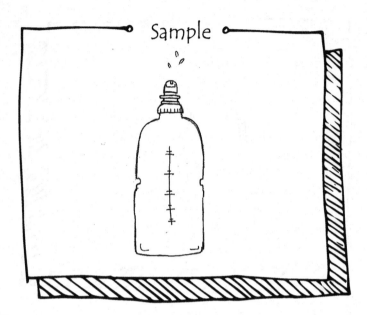

Sample

Consider a doodle of
someone drinking tea

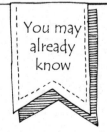

You may
already
know

Polyposia ingesting large amounts of liquids for a long time

Consider a doodle of
P.S. on a letter

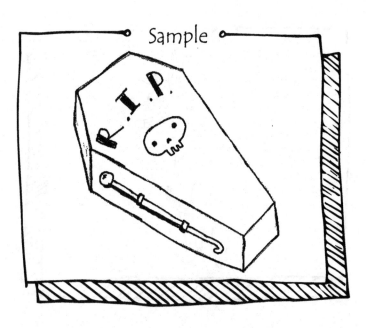

Sample

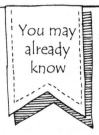

Postoperative after surgery, **Posterior** directed to the back,
Postnatal occurring after birth

Consider a doodle of
a sign on the back of
an animal

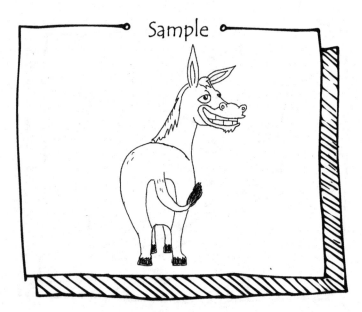

Sample

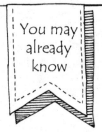

You may
already
know

Posterior directed toward the back, **Posterolateral** situated on the side

Consider a doodle of
a film clip sign

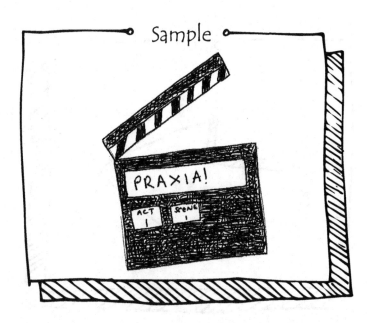

Sample

PRAXIA!

ACT 1   SCENE 1

Apraxia inability to perform purposeful movements, **Dyspraxia** poor movement, **Orthopraxy** mechanical correction of deformities, **Parapraxis** faulty act, such as a slip of the tongue

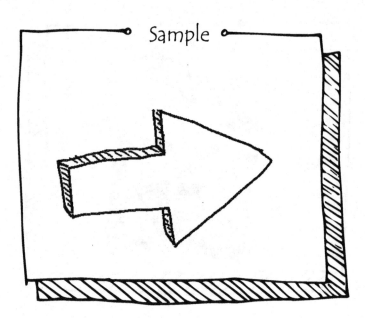

Sample

Consider a doodle of
movie previews

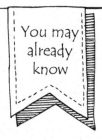

You may already know

Precalculus class before calculus study, **Foreword** section of a book occurring before the main text, **Preset** already arranged, **Preventative measure** a prophylactic, **Preoptic** in front of the optic nerve, **Forearm** part of the arm before the hand, **Premature** before proper time

Consider a doodle of
a prototype machine

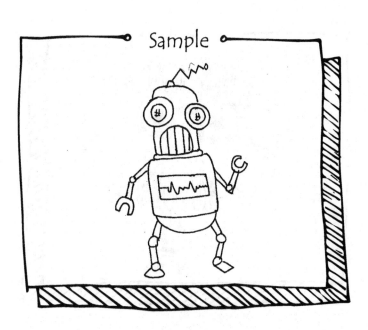

Sample

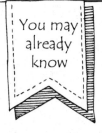

You may
already
know

Profile simple outline, **Prolapse** organ or part of an organ falling down,
Antedate date before finished, **Protocols** first notes of an experiment or report,
Promegaloblast earliest form in abnormal red blood cells

Consider a doodle of
a fake newspaper

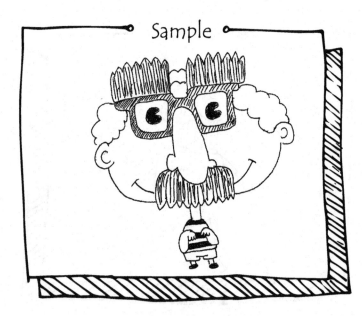

Sample

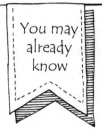

You may
already
know

Pseudonym false name of an author to hide their identity,
Pseudopregnancy false pregnancy, **Pseudoplegia** hysterical paralysis

Consider a doodle of
an itchy arm

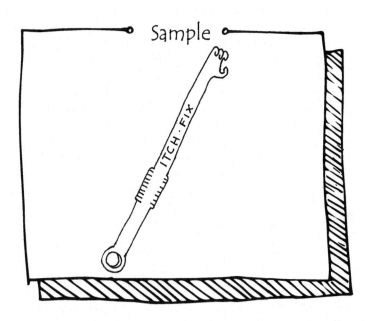

Sample

ITCH.FIX

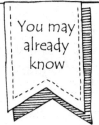

You may
already
know

Psoriasis skin disease marked by red spots and itching, **Psoralen** a plant that causes itching

Consider a doodle of
a tarot card reader or
magic bowl

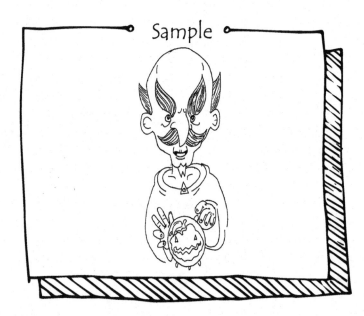

Sample

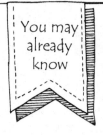

Psychedelic causing abnormal psychological effects, **Psychic** sensitive to
nonphysical or supernatural forces, **Psychopath** unstable person with aggression
and serious irresponsibility, **Psychosis** condition of not being reality bound,
Psychosomatic bodily symptoms caused by mental or emotional reasons

Consider a doodle of
letters drooping down:
P, T, O, S, I, S

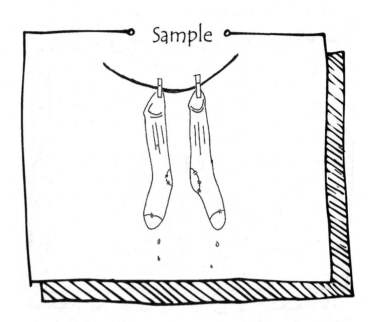

Sample

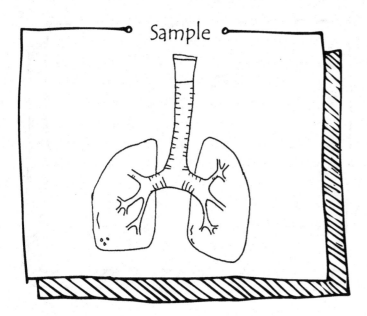

Sample

Consider a doodle of
lungs

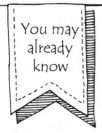

You may
already
know

Pulmonary pertaining to the lungs, **Pneumatic nail gun** a tool used to insert
nails using compressed air, **Pneumatosis** air/gas in abnormal location,
Pulmoaortic pertaining to aorta and lungs, **Pneumonia** inflammation
of the lungs

Consider a doodle of
nails puncturing wood

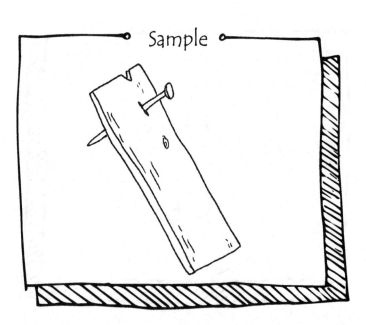

Sample

You may
already
know

Acupuncture alternative treatment involving needles, **Venipuncture** surgical
puncture of a vein

Consider a doodle of
pus-filled letters: P, Y

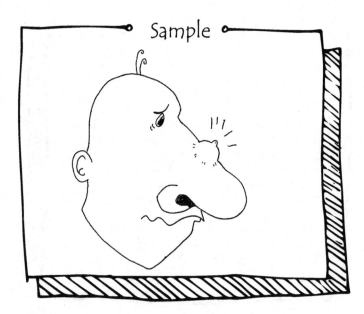

Sample

Pus sac of white blood cells, **Pyorrhea** inflammation of tooth socket with pus

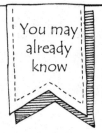

Consider a doodle of
Pyro brand thermometers

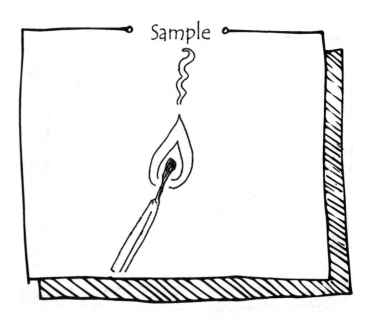

Sample

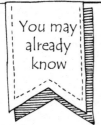
Pyrotechnics a fireworks display, **Pyromania** irresistible urge to start fires

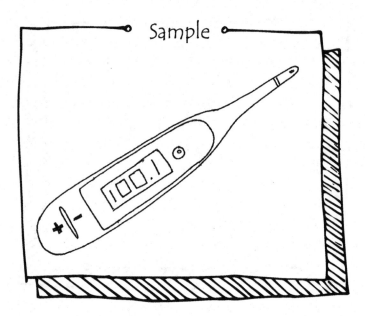

Sample

Consider a doodle of
burning letters:
P, Y, R, E, X

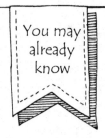

You may
already
know

Pyrex baking dish, **Pyrexia** feverish state

Consider a doodle of
four-leaf clover letters:
Q, U, A, D, R

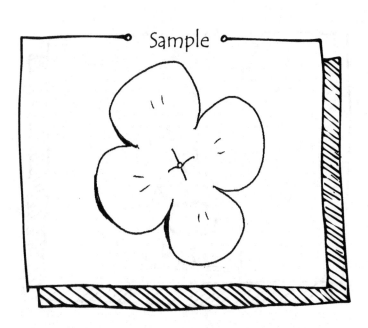

Sample

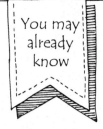

You may
already
know

Quadruplicate four copies, **Tetradactyly** four digits on the hand or foot,
Tetra- or **quadriplegia** paralysis of four limbs, **Quadruplets** four offspring in one
birth, **Quadriceps** four-part muscle group on the front of the thigh

Consider a doodle of
you on the radio

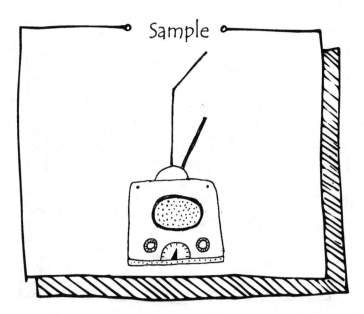

Sample

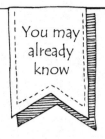

You may
already
know

Radiograph x-ray, **Radioisotope** reactive material

Consider a doodle of
a recycling bin

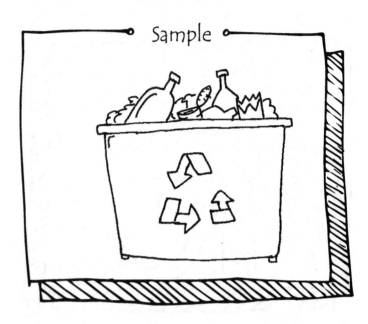

Sample

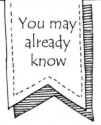

You may
already
know

Rewind to reverse, **Retraction** drawing back, **Recycle** to use again,
Reabsorption absorbing back, **Reflection** thinking back, **Reinforce** to increase
strength, **Regression** returning to an earlier state

- 215 -

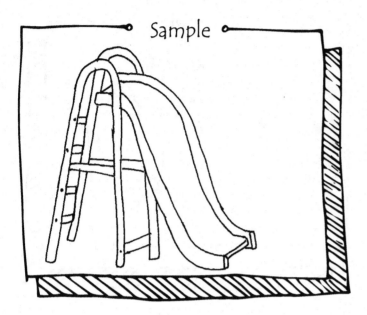

Sample

Consider a doodle of
kids running up a slide
in reverse

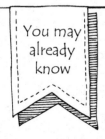

You may
already
know

Relapse to fall back

Consider a doodle of
kidneys

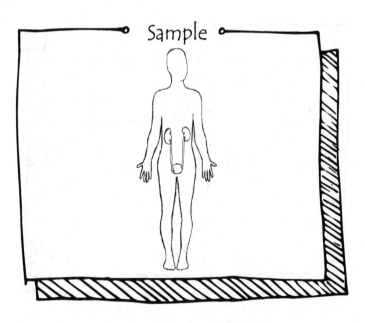

Sample

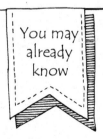

Renal near the kidneys

Consider a doodle of
blowing letters:
R, E, S, P, I, R

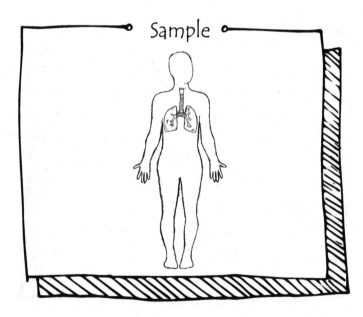

Sample

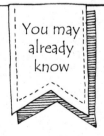

You may
already
know

Respiration process of breathing, **Respiratory therapy** treatment of breathing

Consider a doodle of
a caveman running
backward

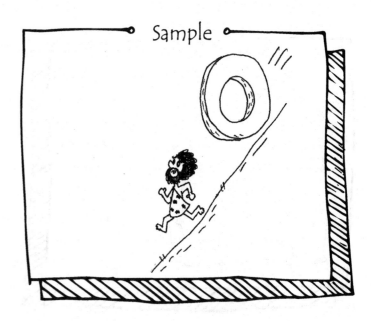

Sample

You may already know

Retro back many years, **Retrodisplacement** moved or displaced backward, **Retrocollic** back of neck, **Retrocolic** behind colon

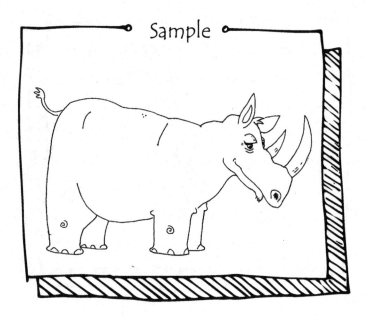

Sample

Consider a doodle of
a rhinoceros

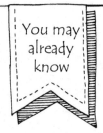

Rhinoceros mammal with a horned nose, **Rhinitis** inflamed nasal passages,
Rhinokyphosis abnormal lump on the nose

Consider a doodle of
drums

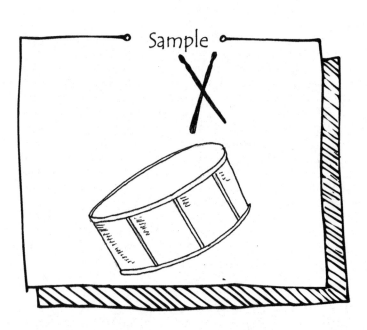

Sample

You may
already
know

Rhythm flow or beat of sound, **Rhythmicity** ability for heart to beat without
stimuli

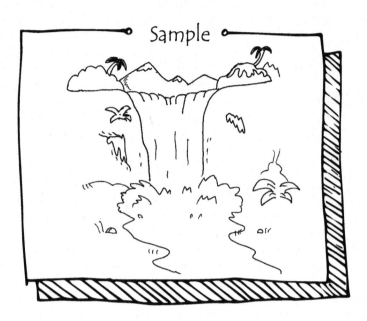

Sample

Consider a doodle of
an exploding island

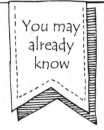

You may
already
know

Diarrhea loose bowel movements, **Stomatorrhagia** hemorrhage from the mouth,
Otopyorrhea purulent discharge of the ear, **Hemorrhage** excessive bleeding

Consider a doodle of
sutured letters:
R, R, H, A, P, H, Y

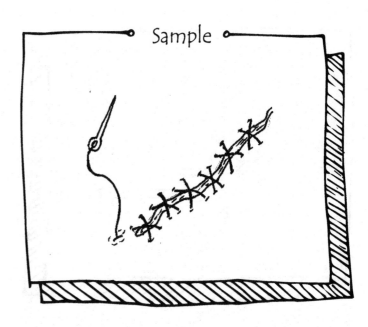

Sample

Myorrhaphy sutured muscle, **Aneurysmorrhaphy** suture of an aneurysm,
Phleborrhaphy suture of a vein

Consider a doodle of
torn letters:
R, R, H, E, X, I, S

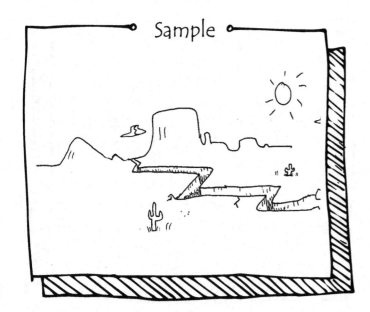

Sample

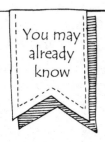

You may
already
know

Myorrhexis torn muscle

Consider a doodle of
hard letters: S, C, L, E, R

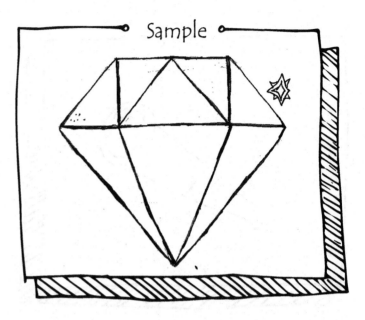

Sample

Scleroderma chronic disorder involving thickening of the skin,
Arteriosclerosis hardening of the arteries

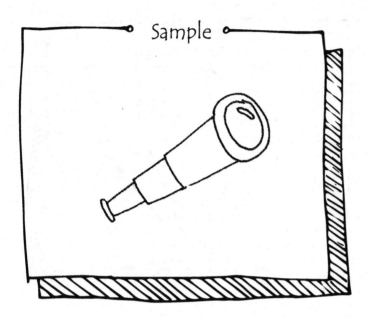

Sample

Consider a doodle of
someone scoping out a
scope

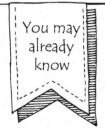

You may
already
know

Stethoscope tool to hear heart sounds, **Microscope** tool to look at small things,
Laparoscopy exam inside the abdomen, **Endoscope** tool to look inside

Consider a doodle of
half of anything

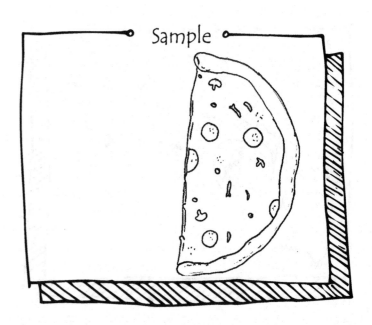

Sample

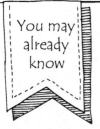

You may
already
know

Semiformal dance with dressy, but not formal, attire, **Seminormal** half the normal strength, **Semicanal** channel open at one end, **Semicoma** stupor

Consider a doodle of
anything sleeping

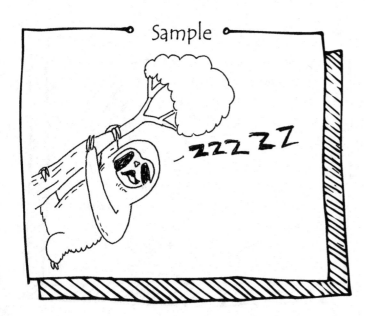

Sample

_zzzZZ

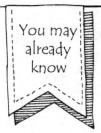

You may
already
know

Insomnia inability to sleep, **Dyssomnia** poor sleep

Consider a doodle of
a hyper kid drinking cola

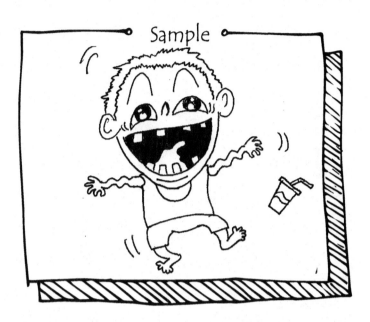

Sample

Muscle spasm involuntary muscle contractions, **Bronchospasm** contractions of
the smooth muscle coating the bronchi, **Myospasm** involuntary contraction of a
muscle or muscle group

- -

Consider a doodle of
an x-ray of the spine

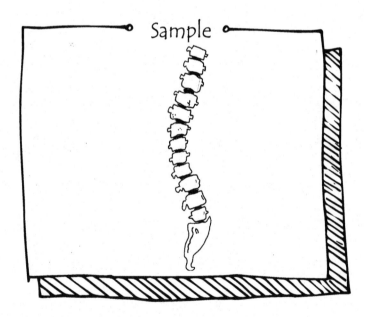

Sample

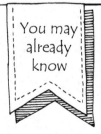

You may
already
know

Spinal pertaining to the spinal cord, **Spondyloarthritis** arthritis of the spine,
Spondylosyndesis a spinal fusion

Consider a doodle of
spongy letters:
S, P, O, N ,G, I

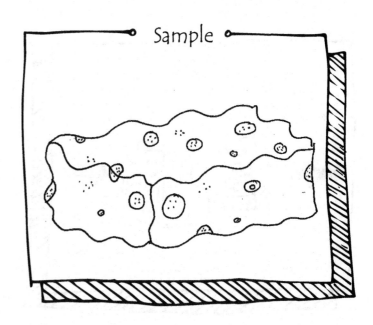

Sample

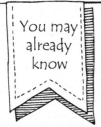
Spongy texture or appearance of a sponge, **Spongiform** resembling a sponge,
Spongioplasm network of fibers pervading the cell substance

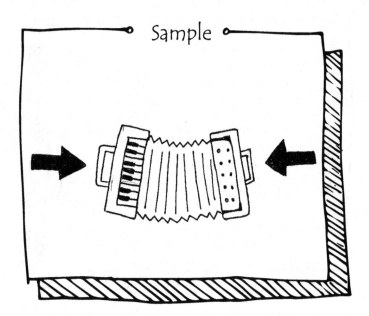

Sample

Consider a doodle of
words that are contractions
(e.g., didn't, couldn't)

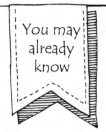

You may
already
know

Static held in position by two or more contractions, **Myotasis** stretching muscle,
Orthostatic standing straight up, **Bradystalsis** slow bowel movement

Consider a doodle of
a scarecrow

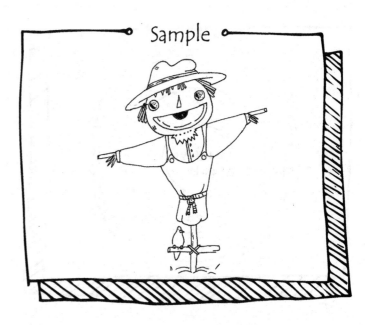

Sample

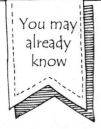

You may
already
know

Homeostasis stable state of being, **Phlebostasis** stopping blood flow in veins

Consider a doodle of
a thermostat

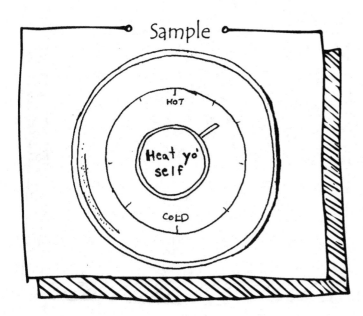

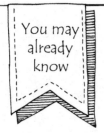

You may already know

Thermostat device to keep temperature stable, **Hemostat** tool to keep a blood vessel from bleeding **Cryostat** device to maintain very low temperatures

Consider a doodle of
hard letters: S, T, E, N

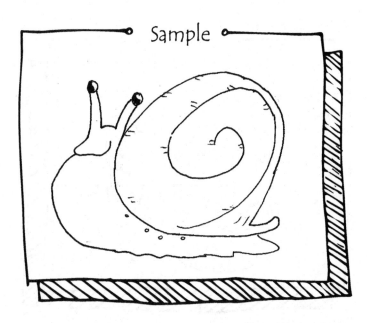

Sample

You may
already
know

Stent device to support tubular structures, **Sclerostenosis** hardening and
constriction combined, **Stenosis** narrowing of a body passage or opening

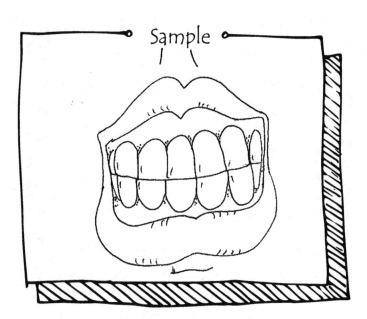

Sample

Consider a doodle of
a mouth eating letters:
S, T, O, M, A, T

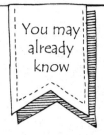

You may
already
know

Stomatopathy disorders of the mouth, **Stomatalgia** pain in the mouth,
Stomatitis inflammation of the oral mucosa

Consider a doodle of
an alien opening a person's
head

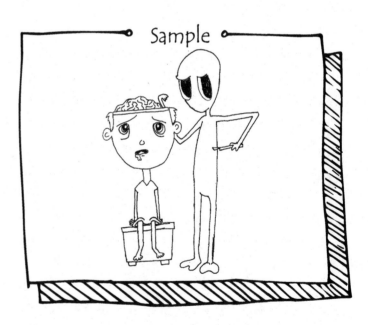

Sample

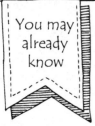

You may
already
know

Stoma bag device to empty the colon, **Phlebophlebostomy** surgically suturing
one vein to another

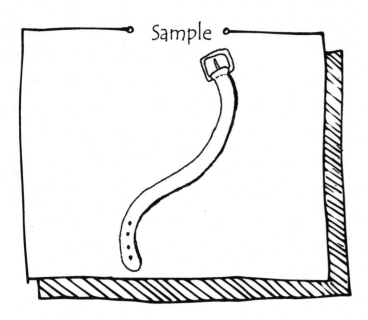

Sample

Consider a doodle of
letters made of belts:
S, T, R, I, C, T

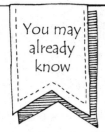

- -

Consider a doodle of
a submarine

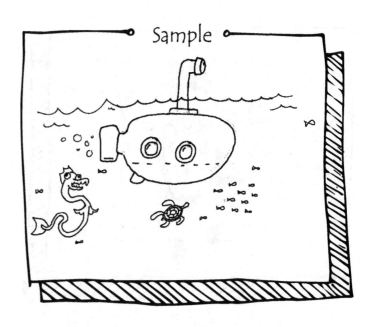

Sample

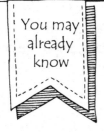

You may
already
know

Submarine ship that can go underwater, **Subzero** temperatures well below freezing, **Subcutaneous** beneath the skin, **Subdural hematoma** blood clot on the brain

Consider a doodle of
a superhero flying

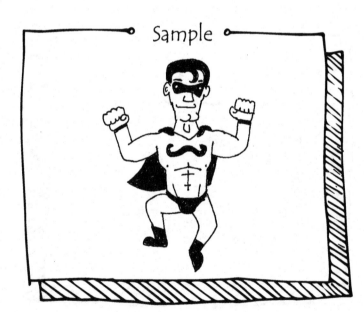

Sample

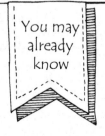

You may
already
know

Superman a hero beyond imagination, **Supernatural** a thought beyond the
natural thinking, **Superficial** on the surface, **Superior** situated above, **Supinate** act
of turning the palm upward, **Superolateral** above and to the side

Consider a doodle of
a supranatural being

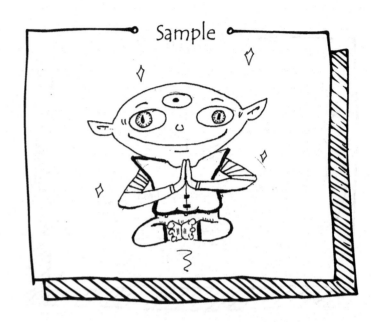

Sample

You may
already
know

Supracostal above or outside ribs, **Supralumbar** above the loin,
Suprarenal above the kidneys

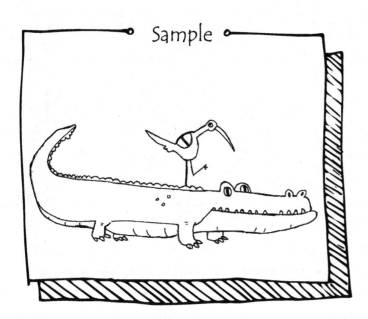

Sample

Consider a doodle of
two animals living together

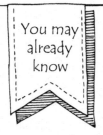

You may
already
know

Symptoms cluster of problems that together make a disorder, **Syndrome** a group
of signs and symptoms that occur together and characterize abnormality,
Synergism interaction of agents or conditions that make a whole greater than
its parts

Consider a doodle of
letters connecting:
S, Y, N, D, E, S, M

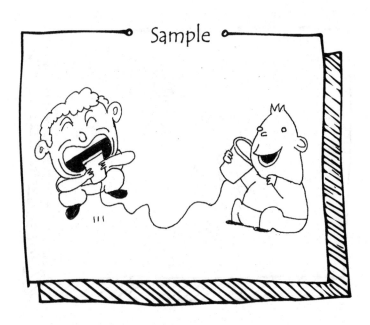

Sample

You may
already
know

Syndesmitis inflammation of ligaments, **Syndesmoma** tumor of connective
tissue, **Syndesmoplasty** plastic repair of a ligament, **Syndactyly** persistent webbing
of fingers or toes

Consider a doodle of
fast-flying stars

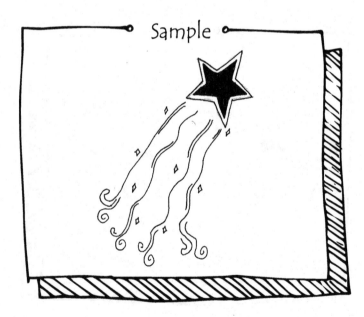

Sample

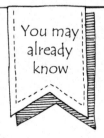

You may
already
know

Tachycardia rapid heart rate, **Tachometer** device to measure speed of rotation,
Tachypnea rapid breathing

Consider a doodle of
cats arranged by size

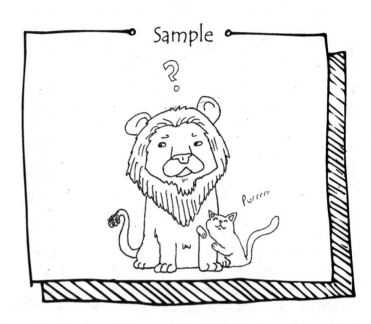

Sample

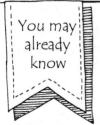

You may
already
know

Taxi arranges transportation for passengers, **Taxonomy** classifies animals by
relationships, **Dystaxia** poor coordination, **Ataxia** without coordination

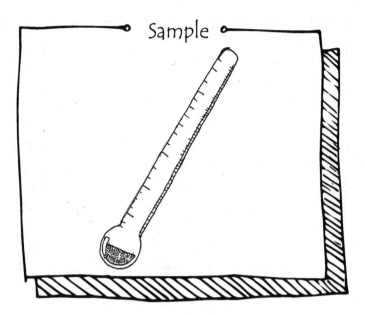

Consider a doodle of
a thermometer

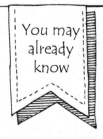

You may
already
know

Thermal pertaining to heat, **Thermometer** instrument to measure temperature, **Thermanalgesis** absence of sensibility to heat, **Thermomassage** massage with heat, **Thermoplegia** heat stroke

Consider a doodle of
a clot blocking a vein

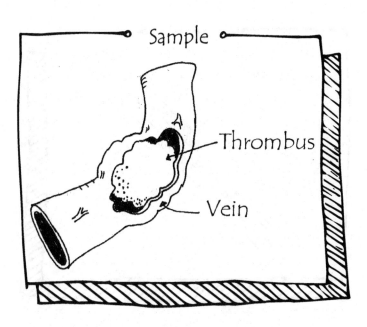

Sample

Thrombus

Vein

You may
already
know

Thrombus mass of blood in living heart or vessels, **Thrombolysis** dissolution
of a thrombus, **Thrombosis** formation of a clot

tom/o, -tome   a cutting (section/layer), instrument to cut

Consider a doodle of
cut out letters: T, O, M, E

Sample

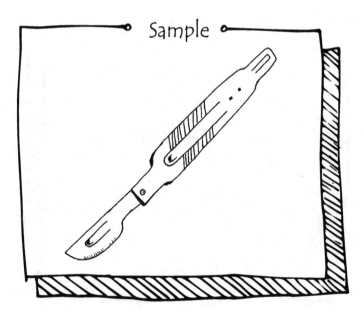

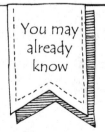

You may
already
know

Urethrotome instrument for cutting urethral structures,
Myotome tool to cut muscle

Consider a doodle of
something to cut out
with the scissors

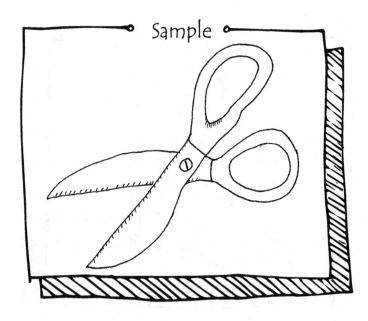

Sample

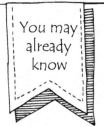
Anatomy dividing the body into areas for study, **Thyrotomy** cutting the thyroid
cartilage, **Celioenterotomy** cut into the abdominal wall to the intestines,
Aneurysmotomy incision of an aneurysm

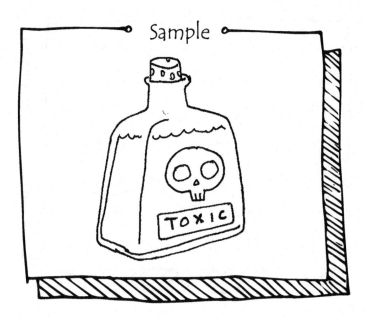

Sample

Consider a doodle of
a bottle of poison

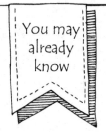

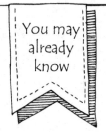
You may
already
know

Toxin a poison, **Toxoplasma** blood parasite, **Toxophilic** easily susceptible to poison, **Urotoxia** toxicity of urine

Consider a doodle of
a bridge to cross

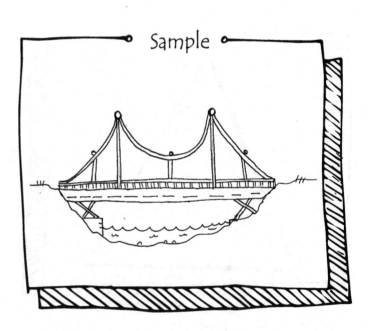

Sample

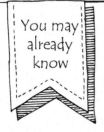

You may
already
know

Transplant or **transport** move from one place to another, **Transfusion** introducing donated blood into the blood stream, **Transgender person** someone whose gender identity differs from the sex they were assigned at birth, **Transference** passage of a symptom or emotion from one to another, **Transfixion** amputation

Consider a doodle of triangles

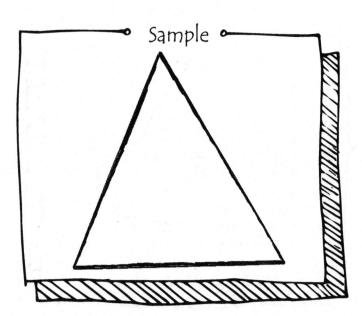

Sample

You may already know

Triangle three-sided shape, **Tricycle** three-wheeled bike, **Triad** group of three related objects, **Triceps** three-headed muscle

Consider a doodle of
a trophy for muscle
building

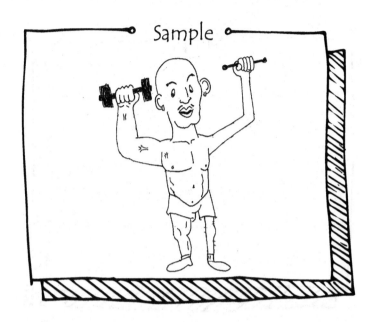

Sample

You may
already
know

Atrophy shrinking or wasting of muscle or organs, **Myotrophic** increasing
weight of muscle, **Myotrophy** nutrition to muscles, **Dystrophy** wasting of muscle
conditions

- 253 -

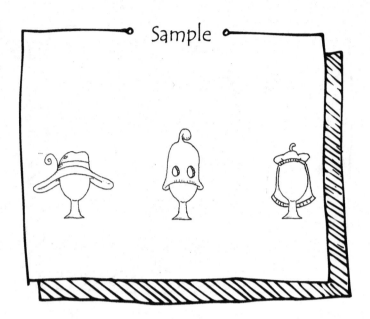

Sample

Consider a doodle of
different types of anything

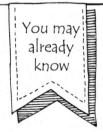

You may already know

Subtype classify types in more detail, **Schizotypal** form of schizophrenia,
Stereotype representative form

Consider a doodle of
excessive food

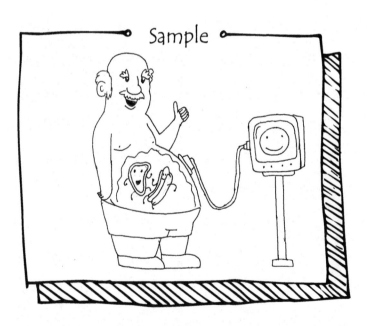

Sample

Ultralight an airplane that is extremely light, **Ultraviolet** violet end of the color spectrum used for treatment, **Ultrasonogram** machine that produces sound to make pictures or heat to provide treatment

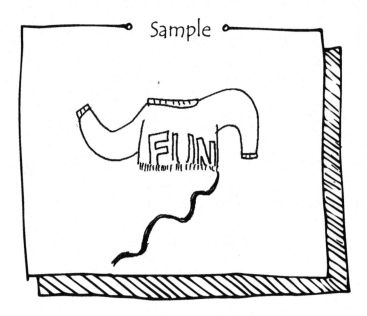

Sample

Consider a doodle of
an undone sweater

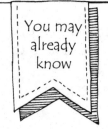

Consider a doodle of
a unicorn

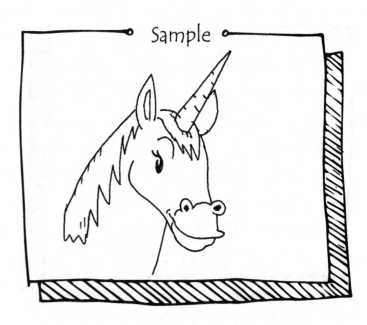

Sample

Unicycle bike with one wheel, **Uniaxial** having one axis,
Unilateral affecting one side

Consider a doodle of
a urinal

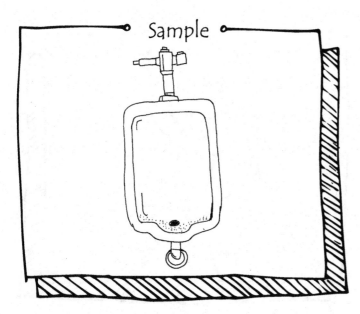

Sample

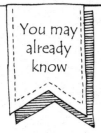

You may
already
know

Urinal receptacle for urine, **Urethritis** inflammation of the urethra,
Uria condition of urine

Consider a doodle of
blood cells in V-shaped
vessels

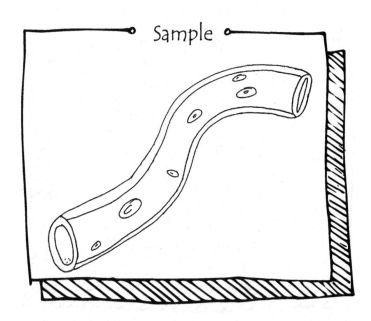

Sample

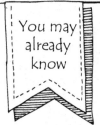
Vase a vessel for flowers, **Vasoconstriction** decreased caliber blood vessels,
Vascular pertaining to vessels, **Vasculature** the vascular system of the body,
Vascularization formation of new blood vessels

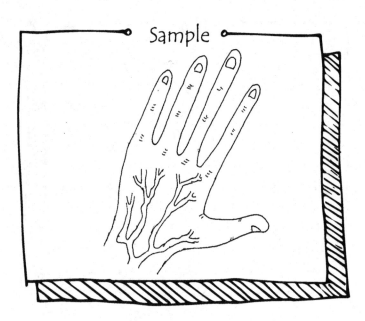

Sample

Consider a doodle of
veins on hands

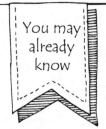

Venn diagram vein or spider-like drawing, **Venation** veins in a leaf system,
Venesection phlebotomy, **Venipuncture** surgical puncture of a vein

Consider a doodle of
bones in the spine

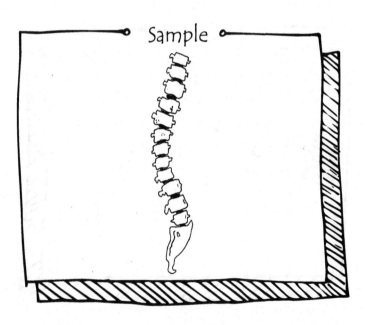

Sample

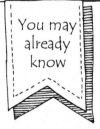

You may
already
know

Vertebrate animal with a spinal column, **Vertebrarium** the whole vertebral
column, **Vertebrectomy** excision of a vertebra

Consider a doodle of
the Grand Canyon

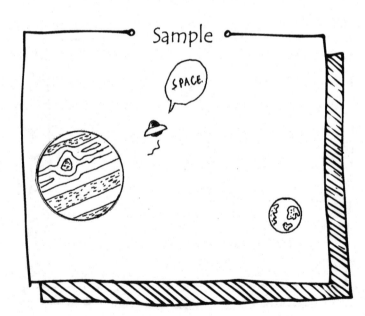

Sample

SPACE.

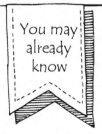

You may
already
know

Vestibule small room on the side of a main room, such as in a church,
Vestibulotomy incision into the vestibule of the ear

Consider a doodle of
virus cells grabbing like
monsters

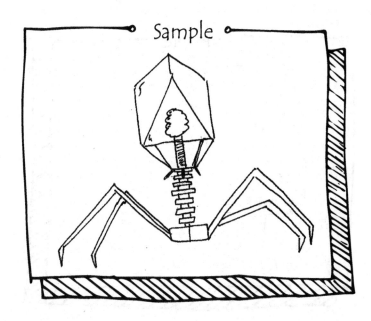

Sample

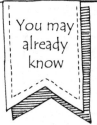

You may
already
know

Viral spread like a virus on social media; caused by a virus, **Virucide** agent that
neutralizes or destroys viruses, **Virulence** degree to which something can enter
host or cause death

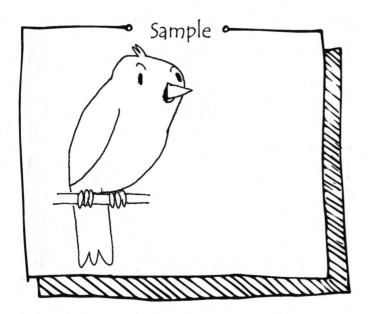

Sample

Consider a doodle of
a yellow bird

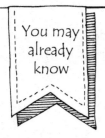

Xanthoma yellow spots on skin, **Xanthemia** yellowing in blood,
Xanthelasma yellow eyelids, **Xanthochromatic** yellow colored, as in
skin or spinal fluid

Consider a doodle of
a dry palm tree

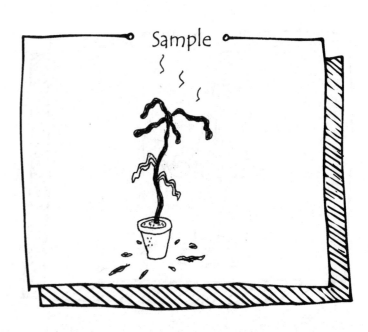

Sample

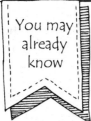

Xerox machine makes dry copies, **Xerophagia** eating dry food, **Xeroma** dry eyes,
Xerocheilia dry lips, **Xeroderma** dry skin

Consider a doodle of
a zookeeper

Sample

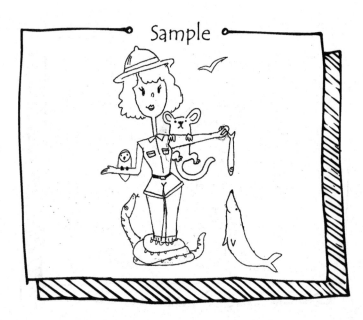

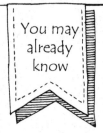
You may
already
know

Zoo collection of animals to visit, **Zoodermic** animal skin used in human skin grafting, **Zoophobia** fear of animals, **Dermatozoon** animal parasite on the skin

Exercises

EXERCISE ONE

JUST FOR FUN ... EXTRA-LONG MEDICAL TERMS

Give the definition for each word provided.

encephalomyeloneuropathy
esophagoduodenostomy
hemangioblastomas
lymphogranulomatosis
oophorohysterectomy
pedisdermatophytosis
periencephalomeningitis
pneumohemopericardium
pneumomyelography
pseudopseudohypoparathyroidism
stereocinefluorography
thermanesthesia
venoperitoneostomy
xanthocyanopsia

EXERCISE TWO

SUFFIXES

Name all the suffixes for:

Pertaining to
Condition of

EXERCISE THREE

COLOR WORD ROOTS

Name all the color word roots.

alb/o
chlor/o
cyan/o
erythr/o
leuk/o
melan/o
xanth/o

EXERCISE FOUR

EASILY CONFUSED WORD ROOTS

Some word roots are naturally confusing. Identify these:

-rrhage

-rrhagia

-rrhaphy

-rrhea

-rrhexis

py/o

pyr/o

-plasty

-ptosis

-pexy

my/o

myel/o

mal-

-malacia

EXERCISE FIVE

SHORT AND TRICKY WORD PREFIXES AND SUFFIXES

Give the definition for each word part provided.

a-

ab-

-ac

ad-

-al

-an

bi-

di-

dys-

epi-

eu-

ex-

hemi-

-ia

-ic

in-

-ism

-ist

-itis

mal-

-osis

un-

EXERCISE SIX

COMMONLY USED WORD PARTS

Give the definition for each word part provided.

a-

ab-

ad-

aer/o

-algia

angi/o

arthr/o

audi/o

auto-

bio-

brady-

carcin/o

cardi/o

-cele

col/o

contra-

crani/o

cyst/o

cyt/o

dent/i

derm/o

-dynia

dys-

ecto-

endo-

eu-

fibr/o

gastr/o

glyc/o

-gram

-graph

hemi-

hem/o

heter/o

hom/o

hydr/o

hyper-

hyp/o

-ic

inter-

intra-

-ist

-itis

kinesi/o

leuk/o

lip/o
lith/o
-logy
macr/o
mal-
-mania
-megaly
meso-
-meter
micro-
mono-
my/o
necr/o
neur/o
-oid
-oma
-osis
ot/o
path/o
-penia
peri-
-phobia
phon/o
-plasty
-pnea
poly-
post-
psych/o
-ptosis
py/o
pyr/o
retr/o
rhin/o
-rrhagia
-rrhea
scler/o
semi-
-stomy
sub-
tachy-
-therapy
thermo/
-tomy
trans-
-trophy
uni-
ur/o
xanth/o

EXERCISE SEVEN

SPECIALISTS

Give the definition for each word provided.

cardiologist
dermatologist
endocrinologist
gastroenterologist
nephrologist
neuropsychologist
oncologist
otolaryngologist
pediatrician
rheumatologist

EXERCISE EIGHT

COMBINED ROOT WORDS

Complete the following sentences:

Destruction or breakup of nerve tissue is _____.

Surgical repair of the ear is _____.

The term for a cancerous growth or malignant tumor is _____.

_____ is difficult or painful movement.

_____ is abnormal fear of fire.

The term for paralysis on one side of the body is _____.

A chronic ailment that consists of recurrent attacks of sleep is _____.

Inflammation of the brain and spinal cord is _____.

A decreased heart rate is _____.

_____ is an enlarged heart.

A term for deficiency of oxygen is _____.

Condition of stiffness is _____.

_____ is herniation of the bladder.

Answer Key

EXERCISE ONE

JUST FOR FUN ... EXTRA-LONG MEDICAL TERMS

encephalomyeloneuropathy	disease of the brain, spinal cord, and peripheral nerves
esophagoduodenostomy	opening between esophagus and the duodenum
hemangioblastomas	vascular ameloblastoma
lymphogranulomatosis	Hodgkin's disease
oophorohysterectomy	excision of the ovaries and uterus
pedisdermatophytosis	athlete's foot
periencephalomeningitis	inflammation of the cortex and meninges
pneumohemopericardium	air or gas and blood in the heart lining
pneumomyelography	x-ray of the spinal cord after air injection
pseudopseudohypoparathyroidism	thyroid condition marked by normal levels of calcium and phosphorus
stereocinefluorography	motion picture camera used in fluoroscopy
thermanesthesia	inability to sense hot or cold
venoperitoneostomy	tool to cut around a vein
xanthocyanopsia	inability to see red or green, vision limited to yellow and blue

EXERCISE TWO

SUFFIXES

Pertaining to -ac, -al, -an, -ar, -eal, -ic, -ive, -ous
Condition of -ia, -ism, -osis

EXERCISE THREE

COLOR WORD ROOTS

alb/o	white
chlor/o	green
cyan/o	blue
erythr/o	red
leuk/o	white
melan/o	black
xanth/o	yellow

EXERCISE FOUR

EASILY CONFUSED WORD ROOTS

-rrhage	excessive bleeding
-rrhagia	hemorrhage
-rrhaphy	suture
-rrhea	flow, discharge
-rrhexis	rupture
py/o	pus
pyr/o	fire
-plasty	surgical repair
-ptosis	prolapse
-pexy	fixation
my/o	muscle
myel/o	spinal cord, marrow
mal-	bad
-malacia	softening

EXERCISE FIVE

SHORT AND TRICKY WORD PREFIXES AND SUFFIXES

a-	no, not, without
ab-	away from
-ac	pertaining to
ad-	toward
-al	pertaining to
-an	pertaining to
bi-	two
di-	two
dys-	bad, difficult
epi-	above
eu-	good
ex-	out
hemi-	half
-ia	condition of
-ic	pertaining to
in-	not
-ism	condition of
-ist	specialist
-itis	inflammation
mal-	bad
-osis	condition of
un-	not, reverse

EXERCISE SIX

COMMONLY USED WORD PARTS

a-	no, not, without
ab-	away from
ad-	toward
aer/o	air
-algia	pain
angi/o	vessel
arthr/o	joint
audi/o	hearing
auto-	self
bio-	life
brady-	slow
carcin/o	cancer
cardi/o	heart
-cele	hernia
coli/o	large intestines
contra-	against
crani/o	skull
cyst/o	cyst, bladder
cyt/o	cell
dent/i	teeth
derm/o	skin
-dynia	pain
dys-	bad, difficult
ecto-	out, without, away
endo-	inside
eu-	good
fibr/o	fiber
gastr/o	stomach
glyc/o	sugar
-gram	record
-graph	recording device
hemi-	half
hem/o	blood
heter/o	different
hom/o	same
hydr/o	water
hyper-	high
hyp/o	low
-ic	pertaining to
inter-	between
intra-	within
-ist	specialist
-itis	inflammation
kinesi/o	movement
leuk/o	white

lip/o	fat
lith/o	stone
-logy	study of
macr/o	large
mal-	bad
-mania	excessive preoccupation
-megaly	large
meso-	middle
-meter	measure
micro-	small
mono-	single
my/o	muscle
necr/o	dead
neur/o	nerve, brain
-oid	resembling
-oma	tumor
-osis	condition of
ot/o	ear
path/o	disease
-penia	deficiency
peri-	around
-phobia	fear
phon/o	voice
-plasty	surgical repair
-pnea	breathing
poly-	many
post-	after
psych/o	mind
-ptosis	prolapse
py/o	pus
pyr/o	fire
retr/o	behind, backward
rhin/o	nose
-rrhagia	hemorrhage
-rrhea	flow, discharge
scler/o	hardening
semi-	half, partly
-stomy	new opening
sub-	under
tachy-	over
-therapy	therapy
therm/o	heat
-tomy	excision
trans-	across
-trophy	nutrition, growth
uni-	one
ur/o	urine
xanth/o	yellow

EXERCISE SEVEN

SPECIALISTS

cardiologist	heart
dermatologist	skin
endocrinologist	glands
gastroenterologist	stomach and small intestines
nephrologist	kidneys
neuropsychologist	brain and mind
oncologist	tumors
otolaryngologist	ear and throat
pediatrician	children
rheumatologist	arthritis

EXERCISE EIGHT

COMBINED ROOT WORDS

Destruction or breakup of nerve tissue is **neurolysis**.

Surgical repair of the ear is **otoplasty**.

The term for a cancerous growth or malignant tumor is **carcinoma**.

Dyskinesia is difficult or painful movement.

Pyrophobia is abnormal fear of fire.

The term for paralysis on one side of the body is **hemiplegia**.

A chronic ailment that consists of recurrent attacks of sleep is **narcolepsy**.

Inflammation of the brain and spinal cord is **myeloencephalitis**.

A decreased heart rate is **bradycardia**.

Cardiomegaly is an enlarged heart.

A term for deficiency of oxygen is **anoxia**.

Condition of stiffness is **ankylosis**.

Cystocele is herniation of the bladder.

Exercises Six through Eight are reprinted with permission from Sladyk, K (ed.). (1997). *OT student primer: A guide to college success.* Thorofare, NJ: SLACK Incorporated.

Medical Terminology Lists

COMPLETE MEDICAL TERMINOLOGY LIST
(WORD PARTS AND DEFINITIONS)

a-, an-	without, not
ab-	away from
abdomin/o	abdomen
acid/o	acid, sour, bitter
acoust/o	hearing, sound
acr/o	extremities
acu-, acut/o	needle, sharp, severe
ad-	toward, near
adip/o	fat
aer/o	air, gas
agit/o	rapidity, restlessness
agora-	marketplace
-agra	severe pain
alb/o, albin/o	white
alges/o	pain sensitivity
-algia	pain
allo-	other, different
ambi-	around, on both sides, about
ambul/o	to walk
ana-	up, backward, against
andr/o	male, masculine
aneurysm/o	aneurysm
angi/o	vessel
ankyl/o	stiff, crooked, bent
anomal/o	irregular
anter/o, ante-	before, forward, front
anti-	against
aphth/o	ulcer
aque/o	water
arch-, -arche	first
arteri/o	artery
arthr/o	joint
articul/o	joint
aspir/o, aspirat/o	inhaling, removal
-asthenia, asthen/o	weakness
ather/o	fatty substance, plaque
audi/o, audit/o	hearing
aur/o, auricul/o	ear
auto-	self
aux/o	growth, acceleration
bacteri/o	bacteria
-basia	walking
bi-	two
bibli/o	books
bio-, bi/o	life, living
blast/o, -blast	early embryonic stage, immature
brachi/o	arm
brachy-	short

brady-	slow
burs/o	bursa
calor/i	heat
carcin/o	cancer
cardi/o	heart
carp/o	wrist
cata-	down, under
cathar/o, cathart/o	cleansing, purging
-cathisia, -kathisia	sitting
cavit/o, cav/o	hollow, cavity
-cele	hernia, swelling
celi/o	abdomen
centr/o	center
cerebell/o, cerebr/o	cerebellum, cerebrum, brain
cervic/o	neck, cervix
chem/o	chemically, chemistry
chlor/o	green
chondr/o	cartilage
chrom/o	color
circum-	around
cirrh/o	orange-yellow
col/o	colon
contra-	against, opposite
cortic/o	cortex
cost/o	rib
crani/o	skull
cry/o	cold
cyan/o	blue
cyst/o	bladder, cyst
cyt/o	cell
dactyl/o	digit (finger or toe)
dent/i	tooth
derm/o, dermat/o	skin
-desis	surgical fixation, fusion
di-	two
dia-	through, throughout
dipl/o	double
dips/o	thirst
dis-	apart, to separate
dist/o	distant
drom/o, -drome	running
-dynia	pain
dys-	bad, difficult, painful
ec-, ecto-	outside, out
-edema	swelling
electr/o	electricity
-emia	blood condition
en-, endo-	inside, within
encephal/o	brain
enter/o	intestines (small intestines)
epi-	above, over, upon
equi-	equality, equal
erythr/o	red
eu-	good, normal, well
ex-	out, away from
exo-	outside, outward
extra-	outside
faci/o	face
fibr/o	fiber, fibrous

flav/o	yellow
flex/o, flect/o	bend
fore-	before, in front
funct/o	performance
gangli/o, ganglion/o	ganglion
gastr/o	stomach
-gen, gen/o, -genesis	production, formation
gluc/o	glucose, sugar
goni/o	angle
-grade	step
-gram	written record
-graph	instrument for recording
-graphy	process of recording
hem/o, hemat/o	blood
hemi-	half
hepat/o	liver
hetero-	different, other
-hexia	condition
homo-, homeo-	same, similar, constant,
hydr/o	water, hydrogen
hyper-	above, excessive, beyond
hypo-	under, deficient, below
iatr/o	treatment, physician
-ician	specialist
inter-	between
intra-	within
-ist	specialist
-itis	inflammation
jaund/o	yellow
kinesi/o, -kinesia, -kinet/o	movement
later/o	side
-legia	reading
-lepsy	seizure
leuk/o	white
ligament/o	ligament
lith/o	stone, calculus
log/o	word, speech, thought
-logist	specialist
-logy	study of
-lysis	dissolution, breakdown
mal-	bad
-malacia	softening
-mania	madness, obsessive, preoccupation
mascul/o	muscle
medi/o	middle
mega-, macr/o	million (10^6), very large number, big
-megaly	enlargement
mel/o	limbs, limb
melan/o	black
meso-	middle
meta-	after, beyond, change
-meter	instrument for measuring
-metry	process of measuring
micro-	one millionth (10^{-6}), small
mi/o	less, smaller
mono-	one
multi-	many, much
my/o, myos/o	muscle
myel/o	marrow, spinal cord

narc/o	numbness, stupor
necr/o	death
neo-	new
nephr/o	kidney
neur/o	nerve
noct/i	night
-noia	mind, will
nutri/o, nutrit/o	nourish
ocul/o	eye
odont/o	tooth
-oid	resembling
-ole	little, small
ole/o, olig/o	oil
olfact/o	smell
-oma	tumor, mass
-opsy	to view
orth/o	straight, normal, correct
-osis	condition, status, abnormal increase
oste/o	bone
ot/o	ear
pachy-	thick
pale/o	old
palliat/o	soothe, relieve
para-	alongside, near, beyond, abnormal
-paresis	partial paralysis
path/o	disease
-pause	cessation
ped/o	foot, child
-penia	deficiency
peri-	around
-pexy	fixation
phleb/o	vein
-phobia, phob/o	fear, aversion
phon/o, -phonia	voice, sound
phot/o	light
physic/o, physi/o, phys/o	physical, natural, nature, air, gas
-physis	growth, growing
-plasty	surgical correction/repair
-plegia	paralysis
pneum/o, -pnea	lung, air, breathe
pod/o	foot
poly-	many, much
-porosis	porous, decrease in density
-posia	drinking
post-	after, behind
poster/o	behind, toward the back
-praxia	action, activity
pre-	before, in front of
pro-	before
pseudo-	false
psor/o	itching
psych/o	mind
psychr/o	cold
-ptosis	prolapse, drooping
pulmon/o	lung
-puncture	to pierce a surface
py/o	pus
pyr/o	heat, fire, fever
pyrex/o	feverishness, fever

quadri-	four
radi/o	x-ray, radiation
re-	back, again
relaps/o	to slide back
ren/o	kidney
respir/o, respirat/o	breathe, breathing
retr/o	backward
rhin/o	nose
rhythm/o	rhythm
rot/o, rotat/o	turn, revolve
-rrhagia, -rrhage, -rrhea	excessive flow, profuse fluid discharge
-rrhaphy	suture
-rrhexis	rupture
scler/o	hard
-scope, -scopy	to view or observe
semi-	half
somn/i	sleep
-spasm, spasm/o	involuntary contraction
spin/o, spondyl/o	vertebrae, spinal column
spongi/o	sponge-like, spongy
-stalsis, -tasis	contraction
-stasis	standing still, standing
-stat	device/instrument for keeping something stationary
sten/o	hardening
stomat/o	mouth
-stomy	surgical opening
strict/o	to tighten, bind
sub-	under, beneath
super-	above, beyond
supra-	above, beyond
sym-, syn-	with, together
synaps/o, synapt/o	point of contact, to join
syndesm/o	ligament, connective tissue
synov/o	synovia, synovial membrane
system/o	system
tachy-	fast
-taxia, tax/o	arrangement, coordination
techn/o	skill, art
ten/o	tendon
tens/o	stretched, strained
termin/o	boundary, limit
tetra-	four
-therapy, therapeut/o	treatment
therm/o	heat
thromb/o	thrombus
tom/o, -tome	a cutting (section/layer), instrument for cutting
-tomy	surgical incision
ton/o	tone, tension
tox/o, toxic/o	poison
trans-	across
traumat/o	trauma, injury, wound
tri-	three
tri/o	to sort out, sorting
-trophy	nutrition of muscles or organs
-type, typ/o	class, representative form
ultra-	beyond, excess
un-	not, reversal
uni-	one
ur/o, urin/o	urine

-uresis	urination
vas/o	vessel, vas deferens
vascul/o	blood vessel
ven/o	vein
vertebr/o	vertebra
vestibul/o	space, cavity before a canal
vir/o	virus
xanth/o	yellow
xer/o	dryness
zoo-	animal

100 COMMON MEDICAL TERMS
(WORD PARTS AND DEFINITIONS)

1.	**a-, an-**	without, not
2.	**ab-**	away from
3.	**acoust/o**	hearing, sound
4.	**acr/o**	extremities
5.	**ad-**	toward, near
6.	**alb/o, albin/o**	white
7.	**alges/o**	pain sensitivity
8.	**-algia**	pain
9.	**allo-**	other, different
10.	**ambul/o**	to walk
11.	**ankyl/o**	stiff, crooked, bent
12.	**ante-**	before, forward
13.	**anter/o**	front
14.	**articul/o**	joint
15.	**-asthenia, asthen/o**	weakness
16.	**ather/o**	fatty substance, plaque
17.	**audi/o, audit/o**	hearing
18.	**auto-**	self
19.	**bibli/o**	books
20.	**brachi/o**	arm
21.	**brady-**	slow
22.	**calor/i**	heat
23.	**cardi/o**	heart
24.	**carp/o**	wrist
25.	**-cele**	hernia, swelling
26.	**chlor/o**	green
27.	**cirrh/o**	orange-yellow
28.	**contra-**	against, opposite
29.	**crani/o**	skull
30.	**cyan/o**	blue
31.	**dactyl/o**	digit (finger or toe)
32.	**derm/o, dermat/o**	skin
33.	**dia-**	through, throughout
34.	**dips/o**	thirst
35.	**dis-**	apart, to separate
36.	**-dynia**	pain
37.	**dys-**	bad, difficult, painful
38.	**ec-, ecto-**	outside, out
39.	**en-, endo-**	inside, within
40.	**encephal/o**	brain
41.	**enter/o**	intestines (small intestines)
42.	**erythr/o**	red
43.	**eu-**	good, normal, well
44.	**ex-**	out, away from
45.	**exo-**	outside, outward
46.	**extra-**	outside
47.	**faci/o**	face
48.	**fibr/o**	fiber, fibrous
49.	**funct/o**	performance
50.	**gastr/o**	stomach
51.	**gluc/o**	glucose, sugar
52.	**-gram**	written record
53.	**-graph**	instrument for recording
54.	**-graphy**	process of recording
55.	**hetero-**	different, other

56.	**homo-**	same, similar
57.	**hypo-**	under, deficient, below
58.	**intra-**	within
59.	**-itis**	inflammation
60.	**kinesi/o, -kinesia, -kinet/o**	movement
61.	**-lepsy**	seizure
62.	**leuk/o**	white
63.	**lith/o**	stone, calculus
64.	**log/o**	word, speech, thought
65.	**-lysis**	dissolution, breakdown
66.	**-mania**	madness, obsessive, preoccupation
67.	**mascul/o**	muscle
68.	**medi/o**	middle
69.	**-megaly**	enlargement
70.	**meso-**	middle
71.	**-meter**	instrument for measuring
72.	**-metry**	process of measuring
73.	**micro-**	one millionth (10^{-6}), small
74.	**multi-**	many, much
75.	**my/o, myos/o**	muscle
76.	**narc/o**	numbness, stupor
77.	**necr/o**	death
78.	**neo-**	new
79.	**nephr/o**	kidney
80.	**noct/i**	night
81.	**ocul/o**	eye
82.	**odont/o**	tooth
83.	**ped/o**	foot, child
84.	**-penia**	deficiency
85.	**-phobia, phob/o**	fear, aversion
86.	**-plegia**	paralysis
87.	**-pnea**	breathe
88.	**poly-**	many, much
89.	**pseudo-**	false
90.	**psych/o**	mind
91.	**psychr/o**	cold
92.	**pyrex/o**	feverishness, fever
93.	**rhin/o**	nose
94.	**-rrhagia, rrhage**	excessive flow, profuse fluid discharge
95.	**-rrhea**	flow, discharge
96.	**-rrhexis**	rupture
97.	**somn/i, -somnia**	sleep
98.	**tachy-**	fast
99.	**-taxia, tax/o**	arrangement, coordination
100.	**tetra-**	four

Printed in the United States
by Baker & Taylor Publisher Services